ANATOMY OF AN EXERCISE CLASS:
An Exercise Educator's Handbook

Carol Kennedy
Deb Legel

SAGAMORE PUBLISHING, Champaign, IL 61824-0673

©1992 Sagamore Publishing, Inc.

Interior design: Susan M. Williams and Michelle R. Dressen
Cover design: Michelle R. Dressen
Illustrations: Deb Legel
Editor: Adrian Hoch
Proofreader: Phyllis L. Bannon

Printed in the United States of America

ISBN: 0-915611-48-1
Library of Congress Catalog Card No.:91-61671

Second printing, August 1992

*This book is for all of the wonderful exercise educators we have worked with
and those we've yet to discover—
And to all of our past, present, and future exercise participants—
you have taught us so much—Thank you!*

CONTENTS

ACKNOWLEDGMENTS

■ We would like to thank the following people for their support, assistance, and most valuable input! Thanks to Darlene Elsea, Deena Luft, and Ted for reading the first draft of chapters 1-3 and offering suggestions and constant encouragement.

Thanks to the exercise physiologists at the University of Illinois (Peggy Gates-Wieneke, Sue Weisel, Susan Bane, and Ellen Evans) for their encouragement and input. To Polly T. Wangman for her discussion, critical review and editing of chapters 1-3 while on holiday and beyond—we owe her a lot! Thanks to Dennis Rewt for his perspective of exercise instruction and sports analysis in a foreign country. To Maureen Ellmore for her ideas, energy, and assistance in developing the first exercise instructor evaluation form.

A big thanks to Lorraine Watts and Joyce Phares for editing the Exercise Instructor Evaluation Tool over and over and over. . . To Deb John (our technical editor), thanks for reviewing and editing the entire book. She added a critical ingredient! To Sara Tutt, R.P.T., Nancy Miller, R.P.T., and Tim Millikan, R.P.T., thanks for their ideas for Chapter 8. Special thanks to Dr. Elliott Plese for his critical review and editing of the entire book. This book really did need his help! We hope that he is as pleased with the results as we were with his assistance!

A big thanks to Marsha Macro for allowing us the opportunity to try out the SEARCH exercise analysis tool at a Rocky Mountain Aerobic Network meeting. To the Department of Exercise and Sport Science at Colorado State University and the Department of Kinesiology at the University of Illinois, we appreciate their belief and support of an academic course on the Techniques of Teaching Aerobics. Much of this information has been taught and reviewed in those courses. To Jim Myers and the instructors at Hewlett Packard in Fort Collins and Loveland, Colorado, our individual evaluation sessions allowed us to thoroughly review and refine the exercise instructors evaluation form and the SEARCH exercise analysis tool. Thanks to Elaine Brush and the Loveland Parks and Recreation Department for asking us to team teach our first workshop together on March 1, 1986 at the old Washington School. This book contains those beginning lecture notes from which our entire handbook was ultimately produced. Finally, exceptional appreciation and thanks to Dann (Carol's husband) for his patience, time with the kids, understanding of our need to publish this information, and recognition that we always had "another project" over the last six years.

INTRODUCTION

■ When we think back to the first exercise classes we taught, we cannot believe we ever instructed that way! The classes consisted of exercises with improper range of motion, little attention paid to muscle balance, and a lack of connection between our workouts and what is necessary for our daily lives. Exercise and exercise instruction have changed immensely in the last 15 years. Considering all of these changes, we were a little apprehensive about publishing our information due to the "in today, out tomorrow" trend in exercise analysis. Yet, over the years, we have come to realize that the human body has not changed; so we decided instead to figure out how we move, why we move, and then how to analyze these movements in the context of our daily routines, jobs and recreational pursuits. We believe this concept is the future trend in exercise instruction.

We have learned that in order for exercise to make any sense we need to understand not only WHAT we are doing but also WHY! For example, do we need to perform 100 outer thigh leg lifts to function more efficiently in our daily lives? Is it necessary to have five minutes worth of abdominal strengthening in every class? These are some of the questions we will address in our book. We know that there are many exercise books that have analyzed specific exercise movements. The purpose of this book is to provide information on safe and effective exercise technique. This includes information on exercise analysis, teaching, cuing, and performing an exercise. We consider the human body's ability to move—what it was meant and NOT meant to do.

This whole process began six years ago when we were asked to teach a seminar on the basics in exercise physiology and how to properly organize an exercise class. That first seminar included many of the principle ideas incorporated into this text, but the general focus has evolved through input from instructors, participants, and our experience.

Our first teaching booklet took more of a cookbook approach with do's and don'ts to be followed. For example, "Do not touch your toes to stretch the hamstrings because this puts stress on the lower back and the muscles are really eccentrically contracting." We were not comfortable with cookbooks or do's and don'ts—they just did not suit our teaching style, nor did they meet the reality of how we run our classes or the vision of what we felt exercise classes needed to be.

We know that the power of exercise is in the process. Every time we teach a seminar, our material changes, and we change. Each time we refine the material, we refine our presentations and our "vision." We want to encourage others to take off their blinders to see that exercise and exercise instruction is NOT black and white, but many shades of gray. For instance, a track athlete who jumps hurdles may need to do the hurdler stretch, however, this may not be a safe exercise for an average exercise participant. Through analysis, we may also discover a better way for the hurdler to prepare for this event.

Could it be possible that increased daily activity (such as taking stairs or short walks throughout the day) can be just as beneficial as your exercise class? Activity versus exercise is one of the "gray" areas that researchers are beginning to study (1,2,3,4). We will discuss how this issue affects the way we instruct our exercise classes.

We believe in the power of exercise to change people's perceptions and their lives.

Exercise is a lifelong process, not an end-product. We want it to have a prominent role in people's lives. We view exercise as one of the last chances that people have in our high-tech, high stress, communication age for self-knowledge, self-expression, personal empowerment, and improvement of health. We want the exercise experience to be exciting, challenging and entertaining, yet safe, healthy and educational.

This book is for those of you who believe that educating your participants is a priority. For many participants, you are his/her first experience with an exercise program since high school. You must strive to encourage participants to become lifetime exercisers by presenting them with a positive experience and educating them about the importance of fitness for a healthy lifestyle. Our major goal in writing this book is to assist you in helping your participants evolve into better people by exercising.

Our book will take you through an entire exercise class with detailed information on organizing a safe and effective exercise session. The first several chapters focus on establishing the attitude and atmosphere of an exercise class, collecting health history information, and considering environment and attire. The remaining chapters will cover the essentials of the warm-up/stretch, aerobic, muscle strength and endurance, cool-down and relaxation segments of an exercise classs. At the beginning of each chapter there will be an outline of the material covered in that segment. We use these outlines when we evaluate individual classes. The entire evaluation tool containing all chapter outlines follows to introduce the book as a whole. We hope you can use this evaluation form as an outline or checklist that will help you teach a better class or evaluate a class effectively.

REFERENCES

1. Monahan, T. Oct. 1987. Is Activity as Good as Exercise? *Phys Sportsmed* 15:10, 181-186.
2. Round Table. Oct. 1987. The Health Benefits of Exercise (Part 1) *Phys Sportsmed*, 15:10115-132.
3. Round Table. Nov. 1987. The Health Benefits of Exercise (Part 2) *Phys Sportsmed*,15:11 121-131.
4. Stamford, B., and Shimer, P. 1990. *Fitness without Exercise*. New York, Warner Books, Inc.

EXERCISE INSTRUCTOR EVALUATION

NAME: _____   EVALUATOR: _____

DATE: _____ CLASS: _____ TIME: _____

SCORING SYSTEM: + = Proficient;   / = Adequate;   0 = Inadequate;   NA = Not Applicable;   NO = Not Observed

ATTITUDE AND ATMOSPHERE CHECKLIST:

Professional Certifications:

____ACSM   ____ACE   ____Other

____ CPR (Expiration Date: _____)

____ Knows Emergency Procedures   _____

Knowledge of Participants' Personal Health:

____ Acquiring health history information   _____

____ Orientation and integration of new participants   _____

____ Available before, during and/or after class to answer questions   _____

Special Considerations:

____ Participant/Instructor Ratio: _____

____ Environmental hazards or conditions addressed   _____

____ Dressed in appropriate footwear/attire   _____

GOAL SETTING --ATTITUDE/ATMOSPHERE: _____

_____

PRE-CLASS ORGANIZATION:

____ Begins class on time (Time started: _____) _____

____ Equipment/tapes ready for use   _____

____ Acknowledges class   _____

WARM-UP STRETCH: _____ MINUTES

____ Beginning segment designed to "break a sweat"_____

____ Range of Motion increased gradually   _____

____ New or complex movements reviewed   _____

____ Major muscle groups stretched in a biomechanically sound manner, with appropriate instructions:

	Warm-Up	Stretch
Quads		
Hamstrings		
Calves		
Shoulder joint		
Others		

____ Muscles kept warm between stretches_____

____ Instructs participants in breathing technique _____

____ Verbal directions clear/music volume appropriate _____

____ Music tempo appropriate for biomechanical movement: _____

____ bpm _____   ____ bpm _____   ____ bpm _____

GOAL SETTING -- PRE-CLASS AND WARM-UP/STRETCH: _____

_____

-over-

AEROBIC EXERCISE _____ MINUTES

- ____ Gradually increases intensity _____
- ____ Maintains intensity while incorporating less stressful movement_____
- ____ Uses variety of impact _____
- ____ Utilizes space appropriately _____
- ____ Uses a variety of muscle groups (especially hamstrings/abductors) _____
- ____ Minimizes repetitive movements _____
- ____ Makes smooth transitions _____
- ____ Promotes independence/self-responsibility _____
- ____ Promotes participant interaction _____
- ____ Emphasizes fun and enthusiasm _____
- ____ Gradually decreases impact/intensity to end aerobic segment_____
- ____ Quads and calves stretched immediately after aerobic segment _____
- ____ Verbal directions clear/music volume appropriate _____
- ____ Music tempo appropriate for biomechanical movement_____
- ____ bpm _____ ____ bpm _____ ____ bpm _____

GOAL SETTING -- AEROBICS: _____
_____

PULSE RATE (PR) OR RATE OF PERCEIVED EXERTION (RPE) APPLICATION:

- ____ PR/RPE charts are on site & visible or participants know recommended THR _____
- ____ PR and/or RPE taken after 6-8 min. of activity; Time(s) taken: _____
- ____ Turns music off for pulse count _____
- ____ Peripheral pulses, excluding the carotid pulse, are encouraged _____
- ____ Participants are kept moving during PR counts _____
- ____ Ten (10) second PR counts are used _____
- ____ Assistance given to participants having difficulty or unusual results _____
- ____ Gives modifications based on PR/RPE results and encourages participants to work at individual levels/abilities_____
- ____ PR not taken too often _____

GOAL SETTING -- PR/RPE APPLICATION: _____
_____

MUSCULAR STRENGTH/ENDURANCE/STRETCHING -- PART 1:

Muscle Group	Position/Exercise for Strengthening	Position/Exercise for Stretching	Comments
Hamstrings			
Gluteus Maximus-Buttocks			
Calves			
Shins			
Lower back			
Abdominals - Rectus			
- Obliques			
Neck			
Quadriceps			
Inner Thigh Adductors			
Outer Thigh Abductors/G. Medius			
Deltoids -- Shoulders			
Latissimus Dorsi			
Rhomboids -- Trapezius			
Pectoralis -- Chest			
Biceps			
Triceps			

MUSCULAR STRENGTH/ENDURANCE/STRETCHING -- PART 2:   _____MINUTES

____ Verbal cues on posture/alignment   _____
____ Encourages and demonstrates proper body mechanics _____
____ Instructs/encourages breathing technique   _____
____ Observes participants' form and suggests adaptations for injuries/special needs _____
____ Corrects/recommends changes in polite, non-threatening way _____
____ Equipment is used safely/effectively (weights, rubber bands, etc.) _____
____ Verbal directions clear/music volume appropriate _____
____ Music tempo appropriate for biomechanical movement _____
  ____ bpm _____   ____ bpm _____   ____ bpm _____

POST STRETCH/RELAXATION

____ Relaxation/energize is emphasized appropriately _____

Post Stretch Muscle Group	Position/Exercise for Stretching	Comments
Hamstrings		
Quads/Hip flexor		
Low back		
Neck		
Shoulder joint		
Other		

GOAL SETTING -- MUSCULAR STRENGTH/ENDURANCE/STRETCHING: _____

_____

"People . . . who arrive at ideas through the brain, without exercising the body, always stay underneath what they think they're on top of."

Pierre Delatire
Walking on Air

ATTITUDE AND ATMOSPHERE CHECKLIST:

Professional Certifications:

- ACSM   ACE   Other
- CPR (Expiration Date:)
- Knows Emergency Procedures

Chapter 1

ATTITUDE AND ATMOSPHERE

THE EXERCISE INSTRUCTOR AS AN EDUCATOR

■   Before we get into the specifics of instructing an exercise class, we need to first address the importance of establishing a positive attitude and atmosphere in your class. When you step in front of the class you are taking on a very important job. The manner in which you go about instructing your exercise class "makes or breaks" the experience for your participants. Who you are, what you value and know, and how you communicate, become evident as you lead your class. You must be an educator! Your attitude must be positive, accepting and caring, knowledgeable, and safe, in order to provide the optimum environment for exercise and personal growth of your participants.

Let's take a minute to look at the "big picture" of why we are even advocating exercise for a healthy lifestyle. According to the American Heart Association's (AHA) 1989 Research Facts (1), more than one in four Americans have some form of cardiovascular disease. The AHA estimated the economic cost of cardiovascular disease to the U.S. in 1989 to be $88.2 billion; this figure includes physician and nursing care, hospital and nursing home services, the cost of medication, and lost productivity due to disability.

A current research study performed at the Institute for Aerobic Research in Dallas has also

shed some new light on the importance of exercise for health. In an eight-year longitudinal study looking at fitness levels and mortality, Steven Blair and colleagues (2) found that the death rates of people with low fitness levels were about twice as high as those for individuals with moderate fitness levels. When people with low fitness levels were compared to those with high fitness levels, the death rates were even greater. Blair concluded that low levels of physical activity and physical fitness are important disease and early death risk factors and are comparable in significance to other well known risk factors such as cigarette smoking, high blood pressure, and high blood cholesterol. Actually, "a brisk walk of 30 to 60 minutes each day" can take a person with low fitness to higher fitness levels and decrease risk of death from heart disease (3).

Back pain is also a major health problem in industrialized countries, and afflicts about 80 percent of the population at some time during their lives. Traditional management of patients with back pain (rest and passive treatment) has not been shown to reduce the length of sick leave or to prevent the recurrence of back pain (4,5). Exercise is being recommended now as a treatment for low back pain (6). In dealing with clients we will be interacting more with physical therapists to establish cooperation so that patients can continue with regular exercise in organized forms (7).

An article in a health education journal discusses how educators are beginning to investigate the opinion that in efforts to mobilize the sedentary individual, too much emphasis has been placed on developing and maintaining cardiovascular fitness. The authors suggest that encouraging low-level physical activity may be the first step in mobilizing the sedentary individual as well as favorably altering his/her heart disease risk factor profile (4).

We also believe it is necessary to acknowledge that about 80% of the population does NOT adhere to a regular program of exercise. The simple fact that most exercise classes are offered for an hour indicates that the fit population is the target group. A half hour class is usually all the beginning exerciser can tolerate. An exercise session of 20-30 minutes which eventually becomes one hour may help us retain more of the 80% of the people who often show up every January for only a few weeks. New research suggests that it may be possible to get the same health benefits from three 10 minute bouts of exercise versus 30 minutes of continuous exercise (5). If changing health behaviors is our goal as educators, it is the beginning exerciser that we need to target. The participant already "hooked" on exercise requires motivation and variety to continue. Your major goal should be to get the beginner excited about exercise. If you focus on and assist the people for whom exercise does not come easily, then you are truly an exercise educator.

Remember that even though research on the importance of exercise is being published in medical journals, our present "health care" system actually accommodates sick people. You as an exercise instructor are helping to prevent disease as well as increasing a person's quality of life. Your job will be increasingly important as the cost of health care rises. We encourage your efforts to educate because you are a vital link to disease prevention in this country. Your role is just as important as the role of health care professionals in educating participants about disease prevention. Since you are a major re-source for people, it is essential that you have a basic understanding of how the human body functions, particularly during exercise. If you are working with special groups (i.e. overweight individuals, pregnant women, older adults, or ill people), then your knowledge needs to be even greater.

THE EXERCISE INSTRUCTOR AS BOTH PERFORMER AND EDUCATOR

■   You play a dual role as an instructor and need to balance the performance aspect of teaching exercise with the educational aspect. Both are equally important. There is a greater likelihood of people coming to you for health information if they enjoy your class and find it interesting and entertaining. This book will focus primarily on the educational aspect of an exercise class because we feel this is the part that has been de-emphasized by our profession, but we also encourage you to attend workshops on motivation, choreography exchanges, and sales techniques to keep the performance aspect of your class motivating and fun.

We have seen our share of "performance" instructors. These types of instructors too often allow their own needs and preoccupations to define the attitude and atmosphere of the class. They usually teach from the front of the room only, correct only those in the first row, and are there for THEIR personal work-out. The "performance" instructor fails to leave his/her ego outside of class and quickly establishes an atmosphere of dependence, intimidation, unattainable goals, and quick fixes.

PERFORMANCE INSTRUCTOR

1. Dependence: *I know the way—do what I do.*

2. Intimidation: *This is an easy exercise; come on, do 10 more! No wimps allowed!*

3. Unattainable goals: *One more week and all those sore muscles will be gone.*

4. Quick fixes: *20 more crunches will flatten those stomachs.*

Let's contrast the "performance" instructor to a "performance educator" instructor. The performance educator strives to establish an atmosphere of independence, encouragement, attainable goals, and reality.

PERFORMANCE EDUCATOR

1. Independence: *Remember to work at your own pace. I will be teaching an intermediate class. It will be your responsibility to monitor your intensity level accordingly. Here's how to. . .*

2. Encouragement: *You're doing GREAT!! Keep up the good work. Remember if there is pain, there will be NO gain. Stay with it, you'll achieve your goals.*

3. Attainable goals: *Learning to exercise regularly is a process that will take time. Adding extra activity outside of class like taking the stairs or mowing your yard will help you reach your goals faster.*

4. Reality: *Abdominal exercises will strengthen your abdominal muscles but will not reduce your spare tire. You must do aerobic exercise to lose body fat. There is no such thing as spot reducing.*

Many of the benefits that people seek from exercise are either elusive or impossible to attain because illusion or negative self-image contradicts reality. Furthermore, the participant may struggle with a values conflict. For instance, if the body your participant wants is a leggy, lithe 5' 10" but in reality he/she is 5' 4", short and stocky, then your participant will never get what he/she desires through exercise. Indeed, exercise will be an experience in failure because the natural aspects of being a healthy, active person are lost.

Value conflicts exist for most of us. There are some things we prize—maintaining health, being slim, looking nice—but we really do not want to have to work hard to achieve these attributes. You as an instructor can negatively reinforce such value conflicts by encouraging fad diets, doing an inordinate amount of floor work or aerobics, or by teaching a "performance" class. We need to instruct participants about the reality of an exercise program.

The reality is that exercise takes time, is work, and all of those "things" you exercise for (health, weight loss, rehabilitation, sports activities) don't come easily. A realistic attitude assumes that "you do not get something for nothing" and sometimes you do not get what you want. This does NOT mean, however, that exercise cannot be fun, wild, exciting, and challenging. You can educate as well as perform— leading your participants through realistic exercise in an accepting and comfortable, yet effective manner. Maintaining the balance between the performance and education aspects of a class is one of the greatest challenges we face as exercise instructors.

Professional Certifications

■   Establishing a positive class attitude and atmosphere must be built on the foundation of participant safety. Safety demands that the instructor has professional certifications that must include cardiopulmonary resuscitation and first aid. Other professional certifications

pertinent to exercise are currently provided by the American Council on Exercise (ACE), the Aerobic Fitness Association of America (AFAA), and the American College of Sports Medicine (ACSM). Many of the certifications involve taking written and practical exams that allow an instructor to demonstrate a basic level of skill in exercise leadership and its related components (i.e., anatomy and physiology, heart rate monitoring, etc.). The ACSM Exercise Leader Certification sessions include an optional workshop to help applicants prepare for the certification examinations. ACSM and AFAA require a written and a practical exam to become certified. ACE currently requires only a written exam. Some companies, recreation departments and health clubs insist that their instructors be nationally certified. Others set up their own training or course work to be completed. Either method is a step toward elevating exercise instructors professionally and also ensures a certain level of knowledge and expertise. But having a certification does not automatically mean that you will be a wonderful instructor. It just means you are serious and willing to increase your knowledge and experience.

We have listed two professional organizations below. Our hope is that one national certification will arise someday from the input of many organizations. Our dream is that the fitness industry will redirect more of the profits from commercial fitness back into the education and certification of exercise instructors. Listed below are the addresses and telephone numbers of two professional certifying bodies.

ACE
5820 Oberlin Drive, Suite 102
San Diego, CA 92121
(619) 535-8227

ACSM
401 W. Michigan Street
Indianapolis, IN 46202-3233
(317) 637-9200

Emergency Procedures

■ An important component of participant safety is that you know and practice emergency drills in case someone experiences a problem during your class. You need to have a plan of action for a variety of emergencies BEFORE they occur! If an emergency or accident does happen, your obligation is to the injured. Many facilities have policies and procedures already in effect that must be followed. While you need to know what those procedures are, you also have to have your own personal plan of action.

Your personal action plan might include:

- Who would be most likely to have trouble in this class and what should I prepare for?
- Be familiar with the contents of the first aid kit and how to use them.
- I stay with the injured person, providing first aid/CPR.
- I assign a member of the class to go get help (occupational health nurse or first aid team) in an industrial fitness program, calling 911 or emergency phone number for an ambulance if necessary, getting other staff members to help.
- I assign a member of the class to begin a cool down for the other participants.
- I identify another class member to help me, if necessary.

If you are teaching classes in churches, schools, or in areas where access to a main office or building is limited, your personal action plan might also include the additional items listed below:

- Know where the nearest phone is.
- If the phone is a pay phone, have change available for an emergency call.
- Know the emergency numbers for medical assistance, police and fire in your community. Have those numbers permanently displayed on or near the phone, as well as addresses, directions to the building and the nearest open entrance. Many commu-

nities use 911, but some communities do not access this system.
- Where is the nearest first aid kit or what equipment should I carry with me?

Hopefully, you will never have to deal with an extreme emergency, and the only person who needs anything from your first aid kit might be a participant requesting a band aid. You still need to be prepared. Outlined below is a real life example of how even a skilled emergency drill can go wrong.

■ *A cardiac rehabilitation program took place in an elementary school gymnasium approximately two miles from a local hospital. This program would stage a mock emergency drill once a month. Staff, participants and responding rescue teams knew the date and time frame of the drill in advance. Class participants were assigned duties. One person would call the emergency number, another would begin a cool down, and a third actually would get to be the victim while the professional staff went through their paces.*

On the night of the scheduled drill, everything was going like clockwork. Charlie "went down," the staff carried out their procedures, Millie began the cool down and Joe dialed 911. Joe became so excited that he could not read the printed information. He was dumbstruck and never relayed the necessary information to the dispatcher. The rescue squad proceeded to trace the call and came expecting a real problem. When they arrived Joe was still holding the telephone receiver.

Practicing drills of this nature would be a good idea, especially if you are teaching a high risk group. Two other aspects of emergency procedures that we would like to share with you pertain to necessary emergency equipment.

We mentioned previously that having a first aid kit would be a good idea. The American Red Cross sells pre-made kits if you do not have the time to make your own. If you would like to organize your own kit, we recommend that you buy your supplies in quantity from your local medical supply company. Putting them in a plastic bag, box or a zippered case would be adequate. The most essential items are listed below:

- 2 or 3 inch ace wrap
- Instant cold pack
- Roll of athletic tape
- An assortment of band-aids
- A pocket mask for rescue breathing in CPR
- Several pairs of rubber gloves

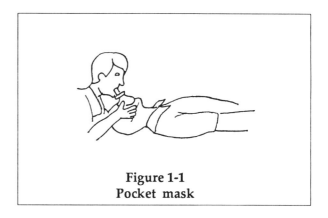

Figure 1-1
Pocket mask

Since the injuries most likely to occur will be cuts, scrapes, strains or sprains, the first four items should handle most of the problems. R.I.C.E.— the acronym for Rest, Ice, Compression, and Elevation— can be used with the first three items on the list.

Swelling after an injury becomes the hardest problem to resolve; therefore, compress the injury with the ace wrap first, apply the instant cold pack, secure it in place with the athletic tape, and elevate the body part on a rolled up mat, towel or jacket. Make sure that your participant gets transported to his/her physician or local Emergency Department for follow-up care as soon as possible. The more time allowed to elapse between first aid and follow-up care, the longer recovery will take. Act immediately!

The last two items on the list concern protecting yourself and your participants from infection and contamination when dealing with an injury, cardiac and/or respiratory arrest or accident.

Any time you are treating an open wound, particularly if there is bleeding, you should put on gloves. Any other bodily secretions should be considered contaminated material and gloves are appropriate protection. The pocket mask for CPR (Figure 1-1) works in exactly the same way. It protects both the participant and the rescuer from cross-contamination.

The pocket mask is a small plastic mask that covers the nose and mouth of the non-breathing victim. A small one-way valve fits into the mask by which the rescuer provides resuscitation. The pocket mask eliminates the need for direct mouth-to-mouth contact and also bars vomitus that might be ejected from the victim during a CPR procedure.

Needless to say, your first aid kit/bag/box must be available in the various exercise areas and shower/dressing rooms. If you are a "traveling" instructor going from place to place, your first aid kit has to travel with you to every class.

To learn the procedures for assessing an injury and how to deal with basic first aid situations, we recommend taking a first aid class from your local American Red Cross Chapter. The Red Cross standard first aid course teaches many quick and simple methods to treat accidents and injuries. It also provides demonstration and practice for adult CPR so you can get two certifications at once. As an exercise instructor, you should be certified in First Aid and CPR. It is your first step towards showing care and concern for your participants.

References

1. American Heart Association, *1989 Heart Facts.* (Dallas, Texas, 1989).

2. Blair, S., H. Kohl, R. Paffenbarger, D. Clark, K. Cooper, and L. Gibbons. 1989. Physical Fitness and All-Cause Mortality: A Prospective Study of Healthy Men and Women, *JAMA,* 262: 2395-2401.

3. *American Institute for Cancer Research Newsletter.* 1990. Issue 28, Summer.

4. Waddell, G. A. 1987. New Clinical Model for the Treatment of Low Back Pain. *Spine.* 12:6320-644.

5. Spitzer, W., LeBlanc, F., Dupuis, M., et al. 1987. Scientific approach to the assessment and management of activity-related spinal disorders. *Spine. 12* (suppl): 75.

6. Cinque, C. 1989. Back Pain Prescription: Out of Bed and into the Gym. *Phys Sportsmed,* 17:9, 185-188.

7. Kellett, K., Kellett, D., and Nordholm, L. 1991. Effects of an Exercise Program on Sick Leave Due to Back Pain. *Phys. Therapy,* 71:4, 283-290.

8. Kasper, M. 1990. Emphasis on Cardiovascular Fitness as a Barrier Toward Mobilizing the Sedentary Individual. *Health Education,* 21:4, July/August, 41-45.

9. DeBusk, R., Stenestrand, U., Sheehan, M., and Haskell, W. 1990. Training Effects of Long Versus Short Bouts of Exercise in Healthy Subjects. *American Journal of Cardiology,* 65:1010-1013.

I begin to see
how a day is adding up,
what I can make of a day,
what a day can make of me.
I begin to see
that I have a choice,
that I can take a hand,
in the design of my everyday.
I begin to see
how I can belong
to me.

Cindy Herbert
Susan Russell
Every Child's Everyday

ATTITUDE AND ATMOSPHERE CHECKLIST:

Knowledge of Participants' Personal Health:

- Acquiring health history information
- Orientation and integration of new participants
- Available before, during, and/or after class to answer questions

Chapter 2

KNOWLEDGE OF PARTICIPANTS' PERSONAL HEALTH

■ How do we go about individualizing and protecting participants during an exercise class? BY KNOWING THE PARTICIPANTS!! You must know where they have been, what they want and need in order to lead them successfully. Knowledge of participants' personal health is an essential part of providing excellent customer service and safety, as well as decreasing professional liability.

ACQUIRING HEALTH HISTORY INFORMATION

■ While there are many ways of obtaining information, a written medical history form filled out and reviewed before a person arrives to class is ideal. Unfortunately, this ideal is often the exception rather than the rule. Using a short medical history form can help solve this problem. All of us have been in the situation where our class is just getting underway when a new participant appears. You can have a new participant fill out the short form upon arrival, quickly review the contents, clarify any vague information and make a mental note of areas possibly needing emphasis during class.

Encourage participants to notify you about changes in their health status or conditions that might warrant modification, even those changes which they may think are small or unimportant. Encourage people to learn as much as possible about their conditions, limitations, or medications. Although it is your obligation to provide a safe work-out, participants also are responsible for their safety and well-being.

Examples of short and long history forms are included for your reference in Appendix A. Please take a moment now to review these forms. These forms have been adapted from many sources and should be changed to fit your specific needs. The format is not really important. What you need is a great deal of information in a small space.

The British Columbia Department of Health designed the Physical Activity Readiness Questionnaire (PAR-Q) to help identify individuals for whom exercise may pose a problem or hazard (1). The PAR-Q could also be used either as a short form or done verbally. If participants answer "yes" to any of the questions listed below, the developers of the PAR-Q suggest that "vigorous exercise or exercise testing may have to be postponed" and that "medical clearance may be necessary." Outlined below are the specific questions contained on the PAR-Q.

1. Has your doctor ever said you have heart trouble?

2. Do you frequently suffer from pains in your chest?

3. Do you often feel faint or have spells of severe dizziness?

4. Has a doctor told you that you have a bone or joint problem such as arthritis that has been aggravated by exercise or might be made worse with exercise?

5. Is there a good reason not mentioned here why you should not follow an activity program even if you wanted to?

6. Are you over age 65 and not accustomed to vigorous exercise?

Another way to get the necessary information is simply to ask questions. Direct questions are the most effective method with latecomers, new participants, or someone in a hurry. For example, we know of an epileptic woman who arrived late for a water aerobics class. The instructor was inserting her musical tape and asked the woman—"Is there anything about YOU or your health that I should know or be aware of?" The woman responded, "I'm an epileptic and had a seizure two weeks ago in another exercise class, so they sent me to water aerobics." "IS THERE ANYTHING ABOUT YOU OR YOUR HEALTH THAT I SHOULD BE AWARE OF?" is about as simple as it gets, but this one question can provide volumes of information.

Sometimes for the safety of the participant you MUST postpone exercise, obtain a physician's release or more information from their health care provider. The American Heart Association (AHA) and the American College of Sports Medicine (ACSM) have jointly published new standards on who needs a medical exam prior to participating in vigorous (defined as $\geq 60\%$ of VO2 Max) exercise (2). ACSM and AHA agree that a medical exam and a physician- supervised maximal exercise test with electrocardiographic (EKG) analysis is desirable for men age 40 and over, and for women age 50 and over. Interpreting risk factors and clinical signs is beyond the scope of this book. We refer you to ACSM Guidelines (1) for futher study. It is your thorough review of the history form that is an essential ingredient in your participants' safety. It is very difficult to turn anyone away from exercise, but you might have to, particularly if the person's history warrants the delay. Be sure to inform the participant of

your concerns and invite him/her to watch your class. Suggest that she/he participate from the sidelines or in the least strenuous activity such as stretching or relaxation. Most programs have physician or medical release forms that make obtaining clearance to exercise the responsibility of the participant.

On the physician release form, incorporate a description of your classes or the activities that the participant might be involved in. Allow spaces for physicians to write in their recommendations and limitations. MOST IMPORTANTLY, if you are dealing with a person with known disease signs and symptoms and/or risk factors, you might have to delay or exclude them from participation. Help him/her find a medically supervised program that will be safe and will meet his/her needs. Discuss your concerns about safety with the participant. Remember, these individuals probably should exercise, but they must be regarded as special people with specific needs. You might not be able to provide the most appropriate exercise for him/her.

Back to our example of the new participant with epilepsy. If, as she states, she had a seizure two weeks ago, her epilepsy is probably NOT under control. She may need to change the dosage of her medication or maybe she is not under a doctor's care. Tell her of your concern and your need for greater information before allowing her to participate; however, invite her to watch the class, introduce her to the participants and occasionally include her in the class banter. When class is over be sure to answer her questions and send her home with a physician consent form. It is important that you do whatever you can to help this person find an appropriate exercise experience.

Once you have medical histories—YOU HAVE TO USE THEM! At the very least you need to acknowledge newcomers and direct specific information at them. For example: "Jim, we do not have very many rules, but since you are new to class, please start slowly, and stop any difficult or painful activity. We will help get you where you want to be, but until you become used to this activity, take it easy!" Also, speak to newcomers during class: "Jim, how are you feeling? If the knee hurts, slow down a bit." Furthermore, don't hesitate to state the obvious when an exerciser may need a "take care" reminder: "Jim, this movement may be very difficult on your knees, so you might forget the side to side movement and just raise your knees straight in front." Finally, remember that other people in the class may learn and benefit from the information given to newcomers. Communicating in this way clearly establishes that the participants' safety and well-being are major concerns of your class.

There are some other problems associated with having all of this information. If you "share" these participants with other exercise instructors, you must also "share" their medical histories and current information. Some system must be developed to exchange this sort of health-related information. Your procedure might be to keep all of the forms in a particular location for all instructors to refer to as needed. Please make sure that a participant's personal health information is kept confidential and is only shared with the necessary personnel. We always make it a rule not to substitute teach in a class in which medical histories and updated information about participants are not provided prior to the time we must take over that class.

ORIENTATION AND INTEGRATION OF NEW PARTICIPANTS

■   Having some kind of health information sheet is the beginning of building a shared responsibility for an exercise class and one way to integrate and orient new participants to your class. To further assist them, provide some written information about exercise, the facility schedule, or the program.

We also want our participants to immediately feel that they are responsible for their work out and for informing us of their personal physical limitations so we can assist them as much as possible. This can be done by having the participant read and sign an informed consent form. A sample of an informed consent form is pictured in Appendix B. Please take a moment to review the form.

We view the informed consent form as ensuring an individual's right to know that there are potential risks associated with exercise. Participants also have the right to know how these injuries may manifest themselves, how the risk of injury will be minimized, and what responsibilities they, as participants, have in avoiding or reducing risk of injury or death.

We use the informed consent form as an educational tool and to introduce the participants to their own health responsibilities in the exercise program. However, use of an informed consent form will NOT prevent a participant from proceeding with a negligence suit against you. The informed consent can be a separate document or combined with a history form.

Both health history and informed consent forms need to be updated periodically. This is particularly important for the history forms. You might ask people to look at their previous form and let you know if there are any changes. How often should you update? At least once or twice a year, or more often as dictated by the needs of the individual.

In summary, it is essential that some type of medical history/informed consent sheet be used. Exercise educators who do not do this are omitting a critical ingredient in demonstrating care and concern for their participants. Also, these forms help establish the foundations of safety, responsibility and communication that are necessary elements of the exercise class.

References

1. American College of Sports Medicine. 1991. *Guidelines for Graded Testing and Exercise Prescription.* Fourth ed. Philadelphia: Lea and Febiger
2. IDEA Foundation. 1987. *Aerobic Dance-Exercise Instructor Manual*, San Diego, 121.
3. Exercise Standards: a Statement for Health Professionals from the American Heart Association, Circulation, 82, 6 (Dec. 1990), 2286-2322.

Now,
now is all the time I'll ever have,
or ever did,
or ever will.
Now is the time
for the creation of now.

I am limited less by
chance and nature
than by my own vision of me.

Cindy Herbert
Susan Russell
Every Child's Everyday

ATTITUDE AND ATMOSPHERE CHECKLIST:

<u>Special Considerations:</u>

- **Participant/Instructor Ratio**
- **Environmental hazards or conditions addressed**
- **Dressed in appropriate footwear/attire**

Chapter 3

SPECIAL CONSIDERATIONS

■   Providing a safe environment is another important responsibility that demonstrates care and concern for your participants. The considerations we will address here pertain to class size, conditions within the exercise area, exercise attire, and perceptions about body image.

PARTICIPANT/ INSTRUCTOR RATIO

■   We have observed 90 to 150 people participating in one exercise class. The instructor usually has a microphone, a podium, and a lot of patience! (It would be interesting to learn whether the instructor knows all of the medical histories of the participants.) We cannot quite understand why organizations/instructors feel that it is necessary to have that many participants in one class. Often it is due to financial gain. These kinds of classes frequently have drop-out rates greater than 50%.

Why? In a large class there is little personal interaction between the participants and the instructor. Physical educators are expressing concern about the lack of interaction in a class (1). Personal interaction among participants and instructors may be our next greatest challenge. Sometimes participants are intimidated by both the podium, the microphone, and probably feel that if they miss a class it will not be noticed. We know of organizations that actually put 90 participants in a class because

they "know" that half of them will drop out. Rather than analyze why these participants are leaving they just accept it. If you have a 50% drop-out rate, please analyze why!

We recommend 20-25 class members in a given class, less if your participants need special care or one-on-one instruction. If you do not know all of the names and histories of your participants, then the class is too big!

In searching for a possible job as an exercise instructor make sure that one of the questions you ask is "what will be the size of the class I will be teaching?" This question may be the most important one in determining how effective or safe you can be. Let's next discuss the environmental concerns of your exercise area.

ENVIRONMENTAL HAZARDS

■   The layout of the exercise area should be free from as many hazards and obstacles as possible.

Examples of hazards or obstacles are:
*   A person walking through the exercise area
*   A fellow exerciser
*   Objects stored in and around the exercise area
*   Equipment (towels, mats, waterbottles) present on the exercise floor

- Fumes from outdoor areas or chemicals being used in an adjacent area
- Pillars or structures within the room itself
- A hot and/or humid room or location
- Inappropriate exercise attire
- Noise pollution (from nearby work areas or music volume that is too high).

Many of the areas that we use for exercise are less than ideal, even those designed specifically for exercise use. Therefore, it is important to inform participants of any hazards or obstacles each time you begin a class as well as any "problem" that may develop during class. For instance, Mary has just entered the class about ten minutes late, she stands at the back of the room and the only place left is between the two pillars that distinguish the exercise equipment area from the aerobic floor. What should you do?

Welcome Mary to class. Remind her that she has missed the warm up and stretching segment and suggest that she stretch her calves, quads, and hamstrings before joining the class. Point out the two pillars and recommend she try another spot or at least be aware of the obstacles. You might even put up signs on the pillars saying CAUTION! DON'T BUMP INTO ME!

Participants should be educated in what constitutes a hazard and told to inform you of any hazards that they recognize. For example, the exercise area is warm and windows have been opened to increase ventilation. One of your participants mentions that exhaust fumes from an idling car in the parking lot are annoying and make it difficult for her to breathe. It is up to you to take appropriate action.

Once again our examples show the fundamental importance of awareness, communication, and the belief that nothing should be taken for granted. Everyone is informed. You should try to eliminate the hazards; and if they are too great, then the class should be moved to another location or cancelled. Your employer and/or building maintenance managers need to be notified of any and all problems with facilities as soon as possible.

ENVIRONMENTAL CONDITIONS

We have talked about environmental hazards. Now let's focus on the actual environment of the exercise area. Environmental factors such as heat, humidity, cold, and high altitude will greatly influence an exerciser's physiological response to exertion.

Heart rates will accelerate with an increase in room temperature (2). If class participants are exposed to heat before arrival or if the exercise area is warm or hot, then heart rates will already be elevated or will increase quickly with exertion. Further increases in heart rate will occur with high humidity. The greater the environmental demands placed on the cardiovascular system, the greater the need for use of target heart rates and/or perceived exertion to monitor the effects of heat and/or humidity on the individual. Participants should be warned that they may reach their target heart rates quicker and may have to modify the intensity of their work out to cope with the existing environmental conditions.

As instructors, we should decrease the intensity of the work out and monitor heart rates often. The duration of the work out should be shorter, water or fluid replacement should be encouraged and if we or our participants notice any of the following symptoms:

1) heat cramps,
2) heat exhaustion; (i.e., dilated pupils, cool, wet, pale skin, body temperature is normal or lower than normal),
3) heat stroke; (i.e., constricted pupils, hot, dry or wet red skin, high body temperature),
4) overall weakness,
5) dizziness, or
6) nausea,

then exercise should be discontinued, and the participant should be moved to a cooler area (3).

If you suspect heat exhaustion or heat stroke you need to get medical assistance for the participant immediately.

Cold is another environmental factor that can affect the physiological response to exercise. In an indoor setting, coolness and cold usually occur because of blowers from ventilation systems in the area. If you have a participant who gets cold easily or may have a condition that is intensified by cold (arthritis, Raynauld's Syndrome, angina, muscle spasms), position that individual away from the source of cold, increase the layers of clothing, have the individual protect affected areas, and keep him/her moving to stay warm. Try to correct the problem in the future, if possible.

If you live in mountainous regions, consider the effects of altitude during exercise. Physiologically, the acclimatization process takes about two weeks. During this time the intensity and duration of a workout must be decreased. Heart rate, blood pressure, and respiratory rate will be elevated to meet the increased demands of exposure and adaptation to higher altitudes. The greater the altitude, the greater the physical demands and the more the exercise period needs to be modified. Even the veteran exerciser will have to curtail activity until acclimatization takes place. Inform your participants about these aspects of modification. Monitor heart rate and breathing rate often. Encourage participants to drink plenty of water to counteract the effects of dehydration from increased breathing rates.

FOOTWEAR

■ Most of us are very aware of the part that good footwear plays in the safety of our participants in exercise classes. Even with the best selection of shoes and some of the best flooring (and there are still many of us conducting classes on linoleum or cement floors), aerobic dance activity takes its toll on both participants and instructors in terms of lower leg injuries. Three separate research studies have verified that over 70% of instructors have or have had an injury associated with teaching aerobic dance exercise classes (4, 5, 6), while another research study found that instructors were twice as likely as participants to be injured during aerobics (7).

Although decreasing impact helps with lower leg injuries, some impact is still present, as is evidenced by the increase in knee injuries related to "low impact aerobics" techniques(8).

Aerobic shoes have been available for a number of years. They provide cushioning (unlike court shoes) and stability for lateral movements (unlike running shoes). Many people still wear either court shoes (tennis, basketball, racquet sports, etc.) or running shoes during an exercise class. Participants should be encouraged to wear athletic shoes that are designed for the specific activity they will be performing. Explaining the rationale behind the requirement usually helps participants understand why they need to comply. Those participants who do not comply may not understand the importance of appropriate footwear. They may feel that they cannot afford aerobic shoes. Try using this example: "Wearing cheap, old, inappropriate footwear during exercise is like having bald, retread tires on a racing car. What you save in tires or tennies you pay for in accidents and injuries. You are doing something good for yourself by being in this exercise class. You deserve new and appropriate footwear."

For the participants who are in many exercise activities, cross-trainers are one solution. (We just wish they had been invented sooner!) Cross-trainers are particularly appropriate if you use interval training, circuits or other exercise equipment in addition to traditional exercise classes.

Once people make a commitment to purchasing good footwear, they are happy. They are so happy, in fact, that they hang on to their exercise footwear far too long. Different shoe manufacturers will tell you various shoe life expectancies, but compression of the cushioning takes place relatively quickly, especially if the people wear their shoes daily and for other activities besides exercise. Rather than put a time limit on the life of a shoe, it is better to look at shoes periodically for signs of wear. Complaints of foot, ankle, calf, shin, knee, hip or low back pain are usually a sure sign that shoes are breaking down.

ATTIRE FOR THE INSTRUCTOR

■   Inappropriate exercise gear worn by an exercise instructor can undermine the best efforts to keep an exercise class non-competitive, positive and healthy. Wearing what fits your style and taste usually works best; however, it is also important to consider the impression, the attitude and atmosphere your personal style conveys. Remember that first impressions are important! We recommend that you use a wide variety of exercise clothing from shorts or sweats to Lycra spandex. Wearing a variety of clothing makes it harder to be labeled and may allow you to appeal to various types of participants. If you share our goal to get as many people as possible exercising, you may get a greater response by wearing a variety of clothing.

We do realize that information and education alone are not what keeps the participants in your class coming back. It is necessary to tap into the feelings and emotions of your participants to create a comfortable atmosphere. The "more revealing" exercise attire can often create an uncomfortable atmosphere for your participants, especially if you have the "perfect aerobic body" they may never be able to achieve. No amount of effort will counter the genetic tendency for some people to have large thighs, buttocks or hips (9).

Psychological researchers have observed that the current fascination with fitness may have the effect of convincing us that "anyone who works out can achieve the lean healthy-looking ideal"(10). Other research notes that women historically have been willing to alter their bodies to match the current societal concept of beauty(11). In the 1990s, the "fit look" is beginning to take the place of the "thin look," especially in the health club scene.

The "fit look" puts an added burden onto the overweight beginning exerciser. In order to belong to the group, he/she needs to lose weight and have a toned body. One study concerning overweight women's perceptions of an exercise program revealed that the most powerful influences affecting their exercise behavior were the concerns about visibility, embarrassment, and judgment by others(12). Thirty-five percent of the overweight participants versus 7% of the non-obese participants dropped out of the exercise program because of social pressure. We do not need to be a certain body type, or look thin and fit to benefit from exercise.

You, as an instructor, can help people become more comfortable with their own bodies and keep them exercising. Wearing a variety of exercise clothing can help facilitate this process.

ATTIRE THAT MAY DECREASE PERFORMANCE AND COMFORT

■   Another safety/comfort issue involving attire concerns clothing with a waist string or belt that is not expandable, which results in constriction of the abdomen. Breathing deeply and from the diaphragm are techniques that increase comfort and capacity during exercise. When exercising, wear expandable, stretchy belts and clothing to facilitate correct air exchange.

References

1. Claxton and Lacy. 1991. Pedagogy— The Missing Link in Aerobic Dance, *JOPERD,* August, 49.

2. American College of Sports Medicine. 1991. Guidelines for Graded Testing and Exercise Prescription,Fourth ed. Philadelphia: Lea and Febiger.

3. American Red Cross. 1988. *Standard First Aid Workbook.* 148.

4. Francis, L., P. Francis, and K. Welshons-Smith. 1985. Aerobic Dance Injuries: A Survey of Instructors. *Phys Sportsmed, 13,* 105-111.

5. Mutoh, Y., S. Sawai, Y. Takanashi, and L. Skurko. 1988. Aerobic Dance Injuries Among Instructors and Students. *Phys Sportsmed,16,* December, 81-88.

6. Richie, D., S. Kelso, and P. Belluci. 1985. Aerobic Dance Injuries: A Retrospective Study of Instructors and Participants. *Phys Sportsmed, 13,* 130-140.

7. Garrick, J., D. Gillien, and P. Whiteside. 1986. The Epidemiology of Aerobic Dance Injuries. *Amer J Sports Med,14,* 67-73.

8. Koszuta, L. 1986. Low-Impact Aerobics: Better than Traditional Aerobic Dance? *Phys Sportsmed, 14:7,* 156-161.

9. Striegal-Moore, R., G. McAvay, and J. Rodin. 1986. Psychological and Behavioral Correlates of Feeling Fat in Women. *International Journal of Eating Disorders,* 5, 935-947.

10. Thompson, J.K. 1990. *Body Image Disturbance Assessment and Treatment.* New York: Pergamon Press.

11. Ehrenreich, B., and D. English.1978. *For Her Own Good; 150 Years of Experts' Advice to Women.* New York: Anchor/Doubleday.

12. Bain, L., T. Wilson, and E. Chaikind. 1989. Participant Perceptions of Exercise Programs for Overweight Women. *Res Q,* 60-2, 1989, 134-143.

"You cannot teach a man anything;
you can only teach him to find it within himself."

Galileo

WARM-UP/STRETCH SEGMENT:

- Beginning segment designed to "break a sweat"
- Range of Motion increased gradually
- New or complex movements reviewed
- Major muscle groups stretched in a biomechanically sound manner, with appropriate instructions
- Muscles kept warm between stretches
- Instructs participants in breathing technique
- Verbal directions clear/music volume appropriate
- Music tempo appropriate for biomechanical movement

Chapter 4

WARM-UP/STRETCH SEGMENT

PRE-CLASS ORGANIZATION

■ Beginning and ending class on time is important. Remember, people have pressing schedules and facilities also are on tightly scheduled time frames. Participants and other instructors appreciate promptness and consideration; therefore, you need to have all equipment and/or music ready BEFORE the class begins. If you do not start on time, this does not necessarily mean you are not a good instructor. If you are addressing a hazard, a safety issue, attempting to assist a class member, or orienting a new participant, you are using time wisely.

Continue to establish your class atmosphere by acknowledging each person's presence. Eye contact, a wave, a welcome and use of a person's name are all part of a positive exercise experience. Immediately orient and integrate any new participants present.

Before starting the class it is important to also acknowledge the class as a whole. Something as simple as "Are you ready? Let's go!" provides the class with an opening. People like beginnings and closures. Use every opportunity to increase your rapport and set a positive atmosphere for the hard work to follow.

Warm-up/Stretch Segment

An effective exercise class starts with the warm-up/stretch segment. If you are using music, the first song you play sets the tone for your class and gets people ready to begin moving. During the first song, movements should warm-up large muscle groups. The second song builds on the first and should permit a combination of warming up and stretching. A class tends to "flow" better if the second song is more upbeat, and the stretching is performed standing so that you can move right into the aerobic segment.

Why Warm Up Before Stretching?

Research has shown that, from a physiological standpoint, stretching a warm muscle is effective and decreases the risk of injury (1). In fact, if we stretch a cold muscle, we can actually do more harm than good. The main purpose of the warm-up/stretch segment then is to generally prepare the body for aerobic activity and stretch the muscle groups that will be used during the aerobic segment to prevent injury. Since we do not know what people have been doing prior to our classes, a warm up is even more essential. Let's look at a real case scenario.

Jean leaves her desk job to come to your 5 p.m. exercise class. She has been sitting most of the day. She wore high heeled shoes to work today; therefore, her calves and hamstrings will be tight from being held in a shortened position. Her back, shoulders, and neck may be fatigued from maintaining a forward posture and perhaps cramped from positioning, alignment, and possible stress. Because she has been involved in resting or sedentary activity, her heart, lungs and diaphragm have been operating at a very low level. Jean arrives at your class and will need the opportunity to prepare her body for increased activity. Her calves and hamstrings, as well as other muscles need to be stretched and lengthened to allow for optimum usage of muscles, tendons, and ligaments during exercise. Her heart and diaphragm, major muscular units essential for aerobic activity, also need to be stretched in preparation for the increasing blood return and deepening respirations. As you can see, the warm up/stretch is a transition between sedentary and vigorous activity and therefore, decreases the risk of injury.

For some of you, the idea of warming up with easy movements and incorporating standing stretches may be a new concept. You may also find it difficult to hold stretches for 20-30 seconds (often suggested in stretching research) and to keep your class from reverting back to bouncing during stretching.

It is our opinion that holding the stretches for the usual 20-30 seconds is not as essential during this initial exercise preparation. Holding stretches for 10-15 seconds is sufficient to lengthen the muscle and supporting structures in preparation for the workout and injury prevention. Holding stretches for 20-30 seconds IS ESSENTIAL AT THE END OF THE WORKOUT, when increasing or maintaining flexibility is our goal.

Ballistic (bouncing) stretching and passive overstretching are incorrect and potentially dangerous. Ballistic stretches have been shown by researchers to be significantly less effective than other stretching methods (2).

Passive overstretching and ballistic stretching initiate a stretch reflex.

Special receptors within the muscle fiber detect sudden or excessive stretching of the muscle. There is a complicated and continual interplay between opposing muscle groups that leads to precision of control and coordinated movement. During this interplay, if a muscle is either activated by a sudden stretch OR continued overlengthening of the muscle fiber occurs, then the system stimulates the muscle to contract rather than lengthen and maintains the contraction to oppose the force of excessive lengthening. Simply put—if you overstretch or bounce and stretch, then the muscle shortens to protect itself. Keep pulling on a shortened muscle and it will either cramp up or rip and tear—but it will NOT lengthen! Thank goodness reflexes are involuntary. If it were not for this stretch reflex, we would have more pulled muscles!

Stretching should be *comfortable* and is encouraged by using cues like "Move to the position where you can feel the muscle pull slightly, then hold; your muscle(s) should NOT feel like a rubberband ready to snap; I know that you can feel the beat of the music, but find a comfortable stretch and HOLD!"

You must also demonstrate stretches without overstretching. If you are a very flexible instructor, you will have to modify how YOU stretch while you lead the class. For example, if you can sit in a straddle position and touch your chest to the ground (Figure 4-1), you are definitely more flexible than the average person; in fact you might be overflexible.

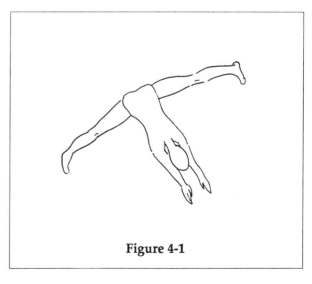

Figure 4-1

For the average person engaging in an exercise class, stretching to this degree is NOT normal, necessary, or desirable. If you lead the stretch like it has been pictured, you can injure someone in your class who is not as flexible as you. Overstretching also gives the person the wrong message (i.e. they should stretch as far as you can). Save the straddle-chest-on-the-floor position for when you visit another instructor's class or when you work out on your own.

A brief note on Proprioceptive Neuromuscular Facilitation (PNF) stretching technique. PNF stretching, for those of you who have not heard of it, consists of isometrically contracting a specific muscle for five seconds, relaxing the muscle for two seconds, and holding a stretch for five seconds, and then repeating this sequence 3-4 times. PNF stretching is based on the principle that muscle relaxation is more profound immediately following an intense contraction.

Current research states that PNF stretching may, in fact, be more effective than the traditional static stretching techniques, particularly for endurance athletes (3). Although this method has proven to be more effective in research studies, we have observed that it is difficult to perform and instruct in a group setting. Advanced exercisers who truly KNOW their bodies and muscle groups, or an exerciser working one-on-one with a therapist seem to benefit the most from this method. Watch for current research on changes in stretching techniques.

Now that we have covered some of the specifics about stretching, let's refer to the Warm-up/Stretch segment of the instructor evaluation form to review the seven important points you should incorporate into your workout.

BEGINNING SEGMENT DESIGNED TO "BREAK A SWEAT"

■ This simply means that before doing any of the stretches you should be warmed up. Methods of warming up should include use of large muscle groups. Moves such as step touches, marching, and hamstring kick backs are a few examples of large muscle movements. How do you know if you are warmed up? You should feel an increase in surface body temperature, particularly in the axillary region (armpits), neck, and hairline. Once you have done this, you are ready to incorporate stretching into your routine.

RANGE OF MOTION INCREASED GRADUALLY

■ When performing the warm-up segment, try to start with smaller moves and increase to larger moves. This allows you to make sure that all of the joints are adequately warmed up in a progressive fashion.

Let's take the shoulder joint for example (Figure 4-2). A progression of shoulder rolls (A), to elbow lifts continuing the circle (B), to a swimming motion using full shoulder rotation (C) would be an effective method of gradually increasing the range of motion of the shoulder joint to provide a safe, effective warm up.

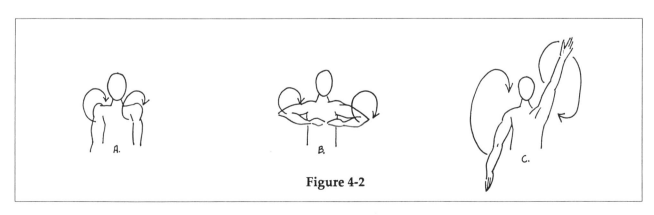

Figure 4-2

NEW OR COMPLEX MOVEMENTS REVIEWED

■   This information applies to your class only if you are using different exercises for circuit training/interval training, or you will be performing aerobic dance or continuous movement routines during your aerobic activity segment. In the cases listed above, you may find that any new participant will tell you that the hardest part of an exercise class is coordination, learning something new or putting new combinations of movements together. Taking the time during the warm-up/stretch segment to introduce a new move or movement combination is ideal. If participants stop often, hesitate or need extra instruction, this is the perfect time to work out the problems. Even if you are not going to introduce a new move, make sure you "get their minds warmed up." Neurons in the brain control what your body does. Patterns are laid down that create the movements that you perform. A move or pattern that was complicated at first becomes easier to remember and execute after practice. Always remember how you felt the first time you attended an exercise class (self-conscious, unsure, ALONE). Realize that there may be someone in your class who possesses all of these feelings. Make sure you warm up both the neuromuscular system as well as the muscles for your new and "regular" participants.

MAJOR MUSCLE GROUPS STRETCHED IN A BIOMECHANICALLY SOUND MANNER WITH APPROPRIATE INSTRUCTIONS

■   We will be discussing the biomechanics of stretching and strengthening by specific muscle groups in Chapter 8. However, let's take a moment to explain why we listed the quads, hamstrings, calves, and shoulder joint muscles with a note that others are optional. These are the major muscles used during the aerobic segment. It is essential to at least stretch these muscles before beginning vigorous aerobic exercise. The inner thigh, outer thigh, and chest muscles also are involved but are not the major muscles used. We are NOT saying that you should ignore stretching these other muscle groups in your routine. Just make sure that the four listed in the evaluation form are ALWAYS in your routine. Rotate others for variety, but never omit the major muscle groups used in the aerobic segment.

MUSCLES KEPT WARM BETWEEN STRETCHES

■   Remember the purpose of the warm-up? Warm up allows the heart, lungs, circulatory system, and muscle groups to prepare for the aerobic activity. When stretching the arm muscles, march, step side to side, perform hamstring kick backs or any other leg movements to keep the legs warm.

Alternating a repetitive movement followed by stretching the same muscle group could be used for the entire warm-up segment. Another example would be to lift your heels for a period of time to warm up the calves, then follow that exercise with a calf stretch. Movement followed by stretching might feel a bit choppy in terms of class flow; however, as far as effective stretching goes, it would be the preferred method.

INSTRUCTS PARTICIPANTS IN BREATHING TECHNIQUE

■   In our earlier warm-up example with Jane, we mentioned the necessity of preparing the diaphragm for exercise. The diaphragm (Figure 4-3) is a domed shaped muscle that separates the abdominal contents from structures of the chest (heart and lungs).

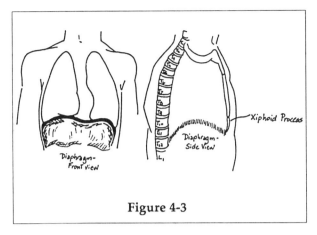

Figure 4-3

The diaphragm is only active during inspiration. Contraction of the diaphragm actually initiates every breath. When the diaphragm contracts it compresses the abdominal contents downward. This action changes the pressure within the chest cavity and pulls air into the nose and mouth. Expiration or exhalation requires no muscular activity. The diaphragm now stretches to its original bell-shaped position.

There are other muscle structures that greatly assist in deep breathing during exercise. The intercostal muscles (muscles between each rib) are major muscles used in breathing. The external intercostal muscles are active during inspiration, and the internal intercostal muscles are active during expiration. Other accessory muscles used during intense breathing are the sternocleidomastoids (prominent neck muscles) and the scalenes (deep muscles of the neck). These muscles attach to the top of the sternum and the clavicle and lift the ribcage during inspiration (4).

All of the muscles used for breathing need to be warmed up before beginning vigorous exercise. You can do this by leading a diaphragmatic breathing exercise (see picture below).

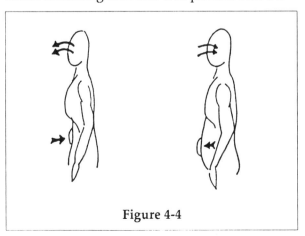

Figure 4-4

1. Start by pulling the abdomen in while exhaling. At the end of the exhalation, you will pause, and inhalation will be initiated.
2. Inhale and allow abdomen to rise; hold the breath.
3. Allow the chest to rise slowly and with control start the exhalation, by—
4. Releasing the chest followed by pulling abdomen in.

Warming up in this way will allow you to slowly increase the rate and depth of respirations and will help participants avoid side stitches during exercise. You know that a participant is working extremely hard to breathe, if he/she complains to you about side stitches or pain at the sternoclavicular joint, or if you notice raised shoulders and prominent neck muscles. Instruct this participant to decrease exercise intensity. Other breathing techniques may also help:

1. Inhaling to a count of four, then exhaling to a count of six will prevent panting and hyperventilation.
2. Exhaling against pursed lips (like you are whistling or sucking through a straw) keeps the small sacs of the lung (alveoli) open longer allowing for greater exchange of gases. More oxygen taken in means increased ability to do aerobic work.

VERBAL DIRECTIONS CLEAR /MUSIC VOLUME APPROPRIATE

■ When explaining what muscles are being worked and how to position the body for optimum effectiveness, it is of utmost importance to speak clearly and confidently. After having evaluated many instructors, we find ourselves constantly reminding them to "tell the participants what muscle is being worked and how to effectively feel the stretch or strengthening exercise." For example, a standing calf stretch is introduced using the following instructions: "Make sure your back toe is pointed forward and your back heel is on the ground. You should feel the stretch in the calf of your leg." Actually point to the calf or touch the participant's calf. "Shift your weight forward onto the front leg to relax the back leg that you are stretching." These are appropriate, effective instructions. If you do not know what to say while leading the specific stretches, refer to the individual muscle group analysis in Chapter 8. Practice the exercise(s) and explanations of what you are doing and why **before** using them in a class setting. If you are truly a professional instructor, you will know what you are doing and let the people know what they should be doing. Remember that the brain controls muscle movement, and the signals to move the muscles originate in the brain. If the participants know what muscles they are stretching, the activity will be purposeful and effective. They will also respect you more as a professional.

Music at an appropriate volume is also a concern we definitely need to address. Exercise classes take place in "open spaces." Other sounds from adjacent exercise or work areas aggravate the noise level even more. All of us know that it is "fun" to crank up the volume and completely envelop ourselves in rhythm, beat and wonderful sounds, but doing so might increase professional liability and health hazards by using high levels of music.

We increase our liability when our music is so loud that participants cannot hear our instructions, warnings, or comments. Imagine a participant on the witness stand. Attorney: "And did the instructor give you instructions so you could avoid getting injured?" Exerciser: "I don't know. I could not hear everything she/he said, because the music was too loud." Check out the back of your exercise area by visiting another instructor's class, or experiment how well you can hear if you are using a piece of exercise equipment. Listen.....can you hear the instructor's directions? Can you hear anything besides the machinery and the music?

Remember, lowering music volume also protects you! Very loud music can damage your hearing and your vocal cords from having to yell over the background noise. You might minimize the problem by circulating through-

out the exercise area and actually become comfortable communicating with the people in your class face-to-face. Perhaps the answer is increasing the number of speakers. What we do know is that the answer is NOT turning up the music or yelling louder.

MUSIC TEMPO APPROPRIATE FOR BIOMECHANICAL MOVEMENT

■ Using an upbeat song during the warm up with strong rhythm to get people going is a good idea. While we want the song(s) to encourage people to "break a sweat," the music should be selected to facilitate the full range of motion of the joints, and slow, progressive movement of the musculature. Music suggested for the warm up should be between 120-135 beats per minute. During the stretching segment of the warm-up period, the music should maintain a steady beat. If you are alternating movements with stretching, you might need to count out loud and/or encourage people to "HOLD the stretching position" even though the background beat is steady or pulsing.

While we have given guidelines for the number of beats per minute of the warm-up/stretch segment, we would like to point out that most of the music we listen to has many rhythms within each song. Some of you (usually those instructors with a dance or music background) can analyze and utilize the different rhythms within a given musical selection. For example, using music with a faster beat per minute count, but utilizing every fourth, eighth or sixteenth count for a particular movement is perfectly acceptable. For those of you with advanced rhythm analysis capabilities, this method works well; however, this technique is NOT for everyone. Rhythms, counting, and cuing are something you need to be very comfortable with. If you cannot get your directions expressed because the tempo is too fast, you will need to slow down the tempo. Find the system that works best for you.

References

1. Eventh, O. and J. Hamburg.1984.*Muscle Stretching in Manual Therapy, A Clinical Manual.* Alfta, Sweden: Alfta Rehab Forlag.
2. Wallin, D., B. Ekblom, R.Grahn,and T. Nordenborg. 1985. Improvement of muscle flexibility-A comparison between two techniques. *Amer Journal of Sports Med, 13:4,* 263-268.
3. Osternig, L., R. Robertson, R. Troxel, and P. Hansen.1990. Differential responses to Proprioceptive Neuromuscular Facilitation (PNF) Stretch Techniques. *Med Sci Sport and Exer, 22:1,* 106-111.
4. Guyton, A. 1986. *Textbook of Medical Physiology.* Philadelphia: W. B. Saunders Company.

A leader is best when people
barely know that he exists.

Not so good when people obey him
and proclaim him,
worse when they despise him.

Fail to honor people,
they fail to honor you.

But a good leader who talks little,
when his work is done,
his aim fulfilled,
they will say—We did this ourselves.

AEROBIC EXERCISE:

- Gradually increases intensity
- Maintains intensity while incorporating less stressful movement
- Uses variety of impact
- Utilizes space appropriately
- Uses a variety of muscle groups (especially hamstrings/abductors)
- Minimizes repetitive movements
- Makes smooth transitions
- Promotes independence/self-responsibility
- Promotes participant interaction
- Emphasizes fun and enthusiasm
- Gradually decreases impact/intensity to end aerobic segment
- Quads and calves stretched immediately after aerobic segment
- Verbal directions clear/music volume appropriate
- Music tempo appropriate for biomechanical movement

Chapter 5

INTRODUCTION TO THE AEROBIC SEGMENT

Lifestyles in Western culture are becoming increasingly sedentary because so many labor-saving devices have been invented to save us time and energy. Elevators, escalators, cars, snowblowers, and electric garage door openers are just a few of these labor-saving products. Many of these inventions save time, but they use energy sources other than our own muscle power. Our participants are encouraged more and more to enjoy convenience-oriented products; however, always remember that when you do, you are choosing to be a couch potato.

You, as an exercise educator, need to remind participants to take the stairs instead of the elevator, to walk to the store when picking up a few items, and to make the choice to physically use their bodies whenever possible. We need to encourage our participants to supplement the exercise class with increased physical activity every day. This is especially true if one of the goals of the participants is weight control.

We know of exercise participants who come to class and drive around the parking lot to get the closest parking space to the building. These same participants usually increase the intensity of their work out to get "more" exercise. We have other participants who choose to walk to class, work moderately, and walk home to cool down. In these examples, the second exerciser demonstrates more appropriate behavior towards healthy living. Our major goal as exercise educators is to convince participants that our class is only a part of their total day and the total health picture. The choices they make

concerning their health and activity levels outside of our classes are just as important as their performance in class. We cannot emphasize strongly enough that exercise will **not** cover all indulgences. Exercise alone is but one of many components necessary for high quality living.

HISTORY OF AEROBIC EXERCISE CLASSES

"Aerobic" means an organism that lives in contact with the air and absorbs oxygen from it (2). You and your participants are "aerobic" organisms. Kenneth Cooper, M.D., was the physician who, in response to the growing numbers of deaths due to cardiovascular diseases, linked the term "aerobic" to activity and disease. Dr. Cooper also devised a well-rounded exercise program that would help people get the exercise and activity they needed to decrease their risk of cardiovascular problems (3).

During the late 1960s and 1970s, exercise, particularly jogging and running, became very popular. People would put on their deck shoes and try running a mile or two often with disastrous results. Many people who could not run, did not like to run, or had been injured from running were looking for alternatives. They liked and believed in the benefits of aerobic exercise and wanted to continue, but running or jogging was difficult, if not impossible. An entire exercise industry was born from individuals who wished to minimize their susceptibility to disease and from those who had experienced looking and feeling better through exercise.

There were many alternatives to running. The most successful by far have been those that were coupled with music. Judy Shepard-Missett developed "Jazzercise". Jackie Sorensen introduced Aerobic Dancing. These programs were just what people were looking for—alternatives to break up the monotony of running and walking, indoor activity for inclement weather, and finally a blend of intense exercise training put to music. Perhaps for many people it met an inner need for connection through participation and movement in a group, very much like folk dancing.

Some people liked the standardized programs of set routines with specific choreography from Shepard-Missett and Sorenson. Other fitness professionals did combinations of calisthenics, dance, and locomotor movements that kept participants moving continuously, but without the necessity of strict form or choreography. This new form of entertaining exercise—this great alternative to running—however, was not without its problems.

In the early to mid 1970s, researchers began to look at whether or not aerobic dance, as it was often called, was a valid form of aerobic exercise. In 1975, Foster concluded that aerobic dance was of sufficient intensity to elicit a training effect and did meet criteria for inclusion in the technical definitions of aerobic activity(4). This research has since been repeated and supported by other researchers using both cross-sectional (5, 6) and longitudinal studies (7,8). However, in the early to mid 1980s, the risk of injury in continuous movement and aerobic dance classes had become an issue.

A 1985 study evaluating clients who had problems associated with aerobic dance concluded that 82% of the injuries were to the lower extremities and occurred after people had begun to exercise vigorously following a period of inactivity(9). Other researchers (10, 11) explored the injury rate among instructors and participants in aerobic dance. Seventy-five percent of the instructors and 50% of their participants were experiencing lower leg injuries. Our own informal surveys at seminars and workshops supported these findings.

Were the participants sustaining injuries because of improper instruction or due to the nature of the activity? Were instructors' injuries due to the frequency of teaching classes, the total duration of time spent teaching, or was the problem a result of the nature of the activity? Was the injury rate high because of rigid flooring, inappropriate footwear, or the nature of the activity? By 1988, the injury rate for aerobic dance participants had decreased   to 22.8%; however, 72% of the instructors were still sustaining injuries (12). Flooring, inadequate footwear, and difficulty in controlling the intensity of an aerobic dance or continuous movement class have all been implicated in the injury rate (13). We also strongly believe that many of the problems are repetitive motion injuries similar to those found in workers who perform the same task repeatedly on a daily basis. Aerobic dance instructors often teach too much and too frequently to allow their bodies, particularly the lower leg, to recover and remain healthy.

During the mid 1980s and early 1990s, the issues of the intensity and impact of aerobic dance activities became the major focus. New class labels were developed: high, moderate and low impact, step aerobics, and water aerobics to name a few.

In high impact aerobics (HIA) just about anything goes; jumping is the norm, and injuries to the lower leg (shin splints and stress fractures) are high. Low impact aerobics (LIA) were initiated as the supposedly "misery-free form of aerobic dance." In LIA one foot remains on the floor at all times to lessen the impact and knee flexion required for shock absorption is emphasized.

The effectiveness of LIA for aerobic conditioning was questioned, since many people had a hard time reaching an aerobic target heart rate (14). Arm movements and hand weights were added to augment the workload. These two factors resulted in more injuries to the shoulder joint, particularly the rotator cuff. The emphasis on shock absorption by the knees led to increased knee injuries. However, LIA was documented to be less stressful on the muscle/joints of the lower leg (15).

Moderate impact aerobics (MIA) were introduced by Lorna and Peter Francis in a 1989 issue of *IDEA Today Magazine* (16). Their concept stressed that one foot remains on the ground so that prolonged knee flexion is avoided. Raising and lowering the center of gravity is used to increase the workload. Other instructors provided mixed format classes by combining high and low impact movement with an emphasis on various kinds of movement across the floor during the high impact segments. A survey (19) done in Australia on aerobic dance injuries concluded that instructors and participants had an injury rate of only 28.9%. Of these injuries, 66% were HIA participants, 9.1% were LIA participants and 7.9% were "mixed" group participants.

We believe that the strictly defined high impact class is definitely a thing of the past. Any activity that injures 25% of the participants is dangerous, indeed, and should be avoided. We also believe that every instructor needs to be able to present various levels of intensity through changes in impact, foot placement, utilization of floor space, and minimization of repetitive movements in EVERY class; therefore, the labels of high, moderate or low impact are extraneous and misleading. We feel that the focus should concentrate on the duration and intensity of effort rather than the level of impact.

STEP/BENCH AEROBICS

■ According to the marketing literature, participants find bench aerobics fun and challenging with less impact and greater benefit. Research studies (18, 19) support the idea that the energy cost for a given individual is dependent upon step height and step rate. The higher the bench, the greater the metabolic cost. Use of hand weights during step aerobics may also increase energy expenditure (20, 21). However, hand-held weights are discouraged because of the risk of injury. **Step Aerobics** seem to be especially attractive to those participants who already are committed to regular exercise and need variety. Currently there is very little research on the risks or benefits of this activity.

Because injuries often appear over a period of years, conclusive research on injury rates with bench exercise is not yet available for true evaluation. An article in *IDEA Today* (22) suggests that some unpublished research has revealed neither any serious injury nor a high injury rate related to step exercise. We are concerned about the potential injury of feet, ankles, and knees. This concern centers on the nature of the activity, which will most certainly produce repetitive motion injury, especially if the participant utilizes the steps for the entire aerobic session or is their only form of aerobic activity. The combination of step and hi/low impact movements seems to be a current trend, and may decrease the risk of the repetitive motion injuries.

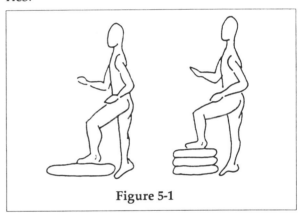

Figure 5-1

WATER AEROBICS

■ Over the last several years, water exercise programs have multiplied at an incredible rate in health clubs, rehabilitation centers, and hospitals. In 1986, there were 500,000 "vertical" aqua exercisers and by 1988, there were 2.2 million estimated the American Fitness Association. In 1990, the number had grown to 4 million and is continuing to rise! We are very strong advocates of water exercise programs because we feel water exercise is bringing in that 80% of the population who would not attend a traditional exercise class or step aerobics class. Water exercise is bringing improved fitness to such a wide variety of exercise participants. From highly trained athletes to participants rehabilitating from hip replacements, water exercise can be adapted to fit any population. Water exercise facilitates movement, conditioning, and strength training in a low to non-impact environment. By making movement easy and by hiding the participant's body, water exercise can minimize the embarrassment and self-consciousness that unfit or overweight exercisers often feel during land exercise (23). Water aerobics does require a special consideration. Movement must be slowed by 1/2 to 1/3 of landspeed for equal energy expenditure (24). Proprioception is different than land exercise. There are several organizations offering educational programs and/or certification in water exercise instruction. Listed below are two organizations to contact for more information:

■   Aquatic Exercise Association
     P.O. Box 497
     Port Washington, WI 53074

     United States Water Fitness Association
     P.O. Box 360133
     Boynton Beach, FL 33436

CROSS-TRAINING— THE BEST AEROBIC ALTERNATIVE

■   Cross-training, the use of many different types of activities to reach and maintain a high fitness level, is the solution to repetitive motion injury and provides the best carryover for sports activities and recreational pursuits. An example of a week of cross-training is outlined below:

Saturday: Water aerobics
Sunday: Brisk walk
Monday: Step aerobics
Tuesday: Rest
Wednesday: Traditional aerobics
Thursday: Circuit training
Friday: Rest

Cross-training is better for instructors because in utilizing different activities they assist and supervise more, thereby reducing overuse of their bodies. Cross-training is better for participants because they receive the benefit of aerobic conditioning (the preparation and maintenance of many muscle groups), thereby optimizing their exercise time and increasing its applicability to their daily lives.

Aerobic activity as defined by the American College of Sports Medicine is that requiring the continuous and rhythmic use of large muscle groups. The exercise must be established at 60-90% of maximum heart rate or 50-85% of maximum oxygen uptake or heart rate reserve. To benefit and strengthen the heart and lungs, these activities have to take place 20-60 minutes, 3-5 days per week (1).

THE SUGGESTED MODE

■   There are many types of activities that are "aerobic" in nature, such as walking-hiking, running-jogging, cycling-bicycling, cross-country skiing, dancing, rope skipping, rowing, stair climbing, swimming, skating, and various endurance game activities. We mention this because we encounter individuals daily who still think that "aerobics" means jumping up and down to music, **not** walking, jogging, cycling, or swimming. The term "aerobics," the phenomenon that has swept American health clubs—where people exercise in a group, performing calisthenics and dance movements to music led by an instructor leaves something to be desired.

Exercise educators have been trying to clarify the definition of "aerobics" to help people understand its usefulness as the major activity to increase cardiopulmonary fitness, an essential component of weight/fat loss, maintenance of bone mass and muscle endurance. We believe that "aerobic" instructors who do not recognize and suggest other aerobic alternatives are only promoting half of the fitness fun at the expense of their customers. We have discussed previously how doing the same thing can lead to injury. Moreover, it can lead to boredom, thus increasing the drop-out rate. Varying the routine allows us to exercise effectively for the rest of our lives.

Use steps, combinations of high/moderate/low impact moves, walking, circuit training, interval training conditioning games and drills (Battleship, soccer/basketball, frisbee). Create an obstacle course, use the pool, and equipment (bikes, treadmills, stair climbers, cross country ski machines). As in nutrition, where variety is the key to success, variety in exercise eases boredom and increases compliance. Can you imagine only eating one food product?

Variety has another benefit. Muscles react very specifically and efficiently to the type of movement and activity they are called upon to do. Runners and walkers perform well on treadmill tests, but not in the pool. Bicyclists score in the high performance category when tested on a bicycle ergometer, but not on a treadmill or in the water. Swimmers do poorly on both the bike and the treadmill. Each exerciser or athlete's musculature is attuned to their method of locomotion. Cross-training, then, allows for greater muscle specificity, because you do not limit the musculature movement, but train to move in different patterns, levels, and intensities.

There is more to "aerobics" than jumping up and down to music. Our Exercise Evaluation Tool looks at the different aspects of leading a safe and effective aerobic segment. Let's look at each aspect in detail.

GRADUALLY INCREASES INTENSITY

■   The human body adapts to exercise very efficiently; however, gradually increasing intensity is necessary to:

1.   Allow blood flow to be redistributed from internal organs to the working muscles.

2.   Allow the heart muscle time to adapt to the change from a resting to a working level. The hardest and most dangerous time for changes in the heart's rhythm is in the transition from resting to high intensity work or from high intensity activity back to resting levels. At rest, the cardio-

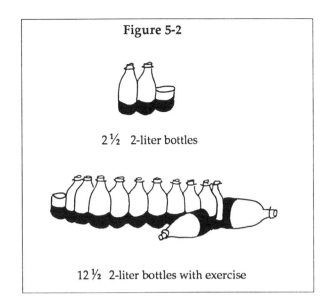

Figure 5-2

2½   2-liter bottles

12½   2-liter bottles with exercise

vascular system circulates about 5 liters of blood per minute. Imagine the contents of two and one half 2 liter soda pop containers circulating through your system every minute. At maximal strenuous exercise, the increase in workload will require as much as 25 liters per minute to accommodate working muscles—that's 12½ pop containers per minute!!

3.   Allow for an increase in respiratory rate. Remember the diaphragm, the major breathing muscle, is like any other muscle and needs time to shift gears. Rapid increases in breathing without time to warm up result in side aches and hyperventilation (rapid, shallow breathing). Some hyperventilation is obviously a part of beginning exercise, but rapid, sudden increases in breathing will increase discomfort and may alter metabolism significantly so that an exerciser cannot continue.

4.   Allow for sufficient warm up (you have begun to perspire), then you do not have to spend precious aerobic activity time warming up further. Your aerobic workout time will be utilized more efficiently.

MAINTAINS INTENSITY WHILE INCORPORATING LESS STRESSFUL MOVEMENT

■   If you are jumping in one place the entire 20-40 minutes of the aerobic segment, you are probably maintaining an adequate intensity; however, it is the constant pounding on the legs that creates many of the overuse injuries of the lower extremities. There are ways to incorporate less stressful movements in any of your programs and to maintain intensity by:

• Instructing participants to use arm **and** leg movements for higher intensities; legs only for moderate intensities; and light, low movements with legs or arms or both for lower intensity.

• Changing the pace of your movements— fast, moderate, slow, ultra slow. Introduce a sequence of movements starting slowly, increasing the speed until the movements are very fast. Let people work at the speed they find most comfortable— monitor heart rates and perceived exertion.

• Changing the size and quality of movement—gigantic, huge, large, medium, small, tiny, heavy, light, strong, weak, staccato, fluid.

• Selecting music that will play a significant role in pacing the size and quality of your movements. It will also create moods through imagery. You might choose fast tempo music but only use every 4th, 8th or 16th beat.

To achieve cardiovascular benefits, the intensity of our workout must remain in our target heart range for a minimum of 20 minutes. The beginning exerciser has the most difficulty with this process. A beginner who experiences failure during the first class will probably not return. Constant reminders are necessary to encourage the beginner to stay at his/her own pace. Leading the class at the beginning level with lots of personal encouragement and eye contact will set the tone and show the beginner how to proceed.

The "hard core" participants have very little difficulty working at a more strenuous pace, but periodically you will have someone request that you work him/her harder. Some instruction on how to achieve greater intensity is always appropriate. We forget to tell our participants that it is also appropriate to maintain a level of exercise that is comfortable. Our participants often feel that they should be going faster, longer, and harder. As instructors, we need to reinforce exercising at a comfortable pace.

Another type of difficult participant to manage is the person who exercises well over his or her prescribed target heart rate and at high levels of perceived exertion. As the instructor you can monitor their intensity of effort by observing the participant's breathing and behavior. For instance, he/she cannot carry on a conversation with you; the person appears dazed and concentrating very hard; or you might see or hear the feet slapping rather than stepping or being placed on the floor. Reinstruct, reinforce, and recheck this person often: explain the purpose of maintaining a specific heart rate intensity and then emphasize this individual's need to monitor his or her heart rate. As an instructor you can also check this person's pulse. A person might be using exercise to gain physical or mental control and might be on a collision course of self-destruction. If you discover this is the case, refer him/her for professional psychological help.

Aerobic Segment as Interval Training

Sometimes the aerobic segment can be taught by using interval training techniques. Interval training allows people to alternate between the hard and easy levels of exercise by working at the higher and lower ends of their target heart rate range (60-90%). However, this does not mean that you alternate between high heart rates and resting levels. If you are using lower intensities of effort, then you need to work longer in order to achieve the same training results. In other words, HIGH INTENSITY—SHORT DURATION and LOW INTENSITY—LONGER DURATION. If you should decide to use these techniques, especially in the aerobic segment, select music that alternates between a fast and a slower beat (for example: 150 beats for the high intensity intervals and 125 beats for the lower intensity intervals).

The ACSM Guidelines suggest that lower intensity over longer durations is more appropriate for adults since there is less likelihood of injury. Newer research also promotes more moderate intensities done on a daily basis as more beneficial for health maintenance and weight reduction (25, 26).

USES VARIETY OF IMPACT

■   We must emphasize the importance of using different locomotor movements in the aerobic segment. A class composed of different types of jumping will be dangerous for both participants and instructors. Below is an example of how to vary the impact pattern:

- Two-step forward, 8 counts (moderate impact)

- Four standing knee lifts with a half turn, face back of exercise area (low impact)

- Jog forward, 8 counts (high impact)

- Four standing knee lifts with a half turn, face front of exercise area (low impact).

A review of basic locomotor skills may also help you liven up your classes and allow you to identify high/moderate/low impact moves. Locomotor movements are those that get you from one place to another. The movements will be listed in order of progression of impact (L=low; M=moderate; H=high). When necessary, we have described the locomotor movement so that we are all thinking of the same activity.

(L) Walking—the most efficient mode of locomotion, the mainstay of low impact movement; easily used daily by most people.

(M) Marching—Walking with knees lifted.

(H) Jogging or Running—For split seconds of time, both feet are off the ground. Jogging can be higher impact since there is less forward momentum and more up and down movement.

(L) Sliding—Step-together-step, both feet remain on the floor. Movement can go forward, backward, side to side, or diagonally.

(M) or (H) Galloping—Step-together-step with same foot leading and with both feet leaving the floor.

(H) Hopping—leaving the floor with one foot or two, landing on one foot only in the same spot. Full body weight is coming down on one foot.

(H) Jumping—Leaving the floor with both feet, landing on two feet either apart or together. Full body weight is coming down on both feet.

(H) Leaping—Same as hopping, but landing on one foot in a different spot most often with one foot forward, and one foot back.

(M) or (H) Skipping—a combination of stepping, hopping or leaping depending on distance covered.

We use the above movements as a foundation to build combinations because they are basic movement patterns everyone was taught in grade school. Some of the new "funk aerobics" and hip gyrations can be fun, but may take the average person some time to feel comfortable. While we suggest using a variety of locomotor movements, please be aware that even locomotor movements can be very hard on the lower legs and back, particularly if you are moving your class across the floor. Jumping, hopping, leaping and skipping are NOT for everyone and alternative movements must always be provided.

Make sure that you instruct your participants on proper landing. The knees should be unlocked or bent on landing so the quadricep muscles can absorb the shock. Pictured in Figure 5-3 is an example of how you can modify the landing in a jumping jack to allow the quadriceps to absorb much of the shock, thereby protecting the knees and low back. This is even true when jumping up and down in water where the body weight is minimized. This position is what we mean when we say the knees need to be unlocked or bent on any landing (Figure 5-3).

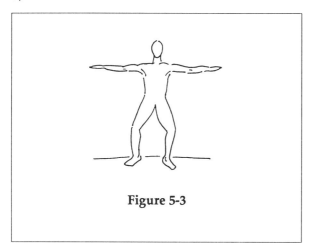

Figure 5-3

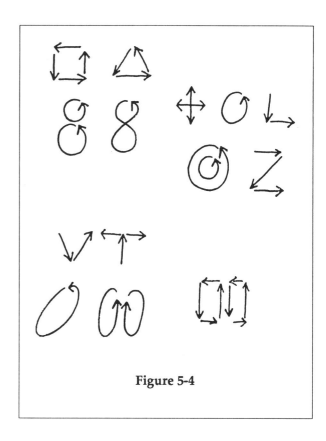

Figure 5-4

UTILIZES SPACE APPROPRIATELY

■ Make the most of your floor space, however limited, and use different geometric configurations during the aerobic segment to help increase safety and interest. Smaller areas often require that you perform exercises in a limited space that often leads to jumping movements; then you are right back to the injury and uninteresting "treadmill" again.

Larger spaces allow you to walk, skip, gallop and use large locomotor patterns more effectively; however, many of the following patterns will give you some idea of what you can do even in a small space. Use of floor space and use of changing patterns is a method of preventing injury and creating a more interesting exercise session (Figure 5-4).

USES A VARIETY OF MUSCLE GROUPS (ESPECIALLY HAMSTRINGS/ ABDUCTORS)

■ We use our quadriceps and hip flexor muscle groups a great deal during our daily activities. Some individuals, because of the nature of their work and lifestyles, use these two muscle groups almost exclusively; therefore, continuing to use the quadriceps and hip flexors repeatedly during exercise is unnecessary. We must balance daily flexion with other movements, for instance hamstring and abductor work.

Keeping the hip extended/straight, pointing the knee towards the ground, and bringing the foot off of the ground will stretch the flexors and work the hamstring group. Moving the legs from side to side will work abductor and adductor groups (Figure 5-5).

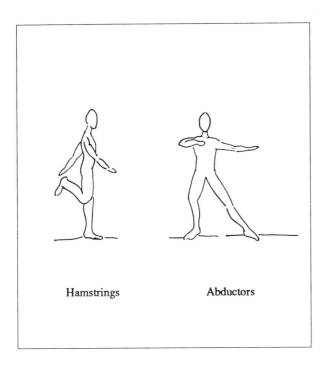

Hamstrings   Abductors

Figure 5-5

Below are suggestions for using various muscle groups:

• Use movement combinations and choreography (step-together-step; step right, cross over left, step right . . .).

• Use different levels—high (on toes, arms up overhead), medium, low and everything in between.

• Mix foot patterns—4 heel touches, 4 toe touches or heel-toe, slide, slide, heel-toe, slide. . .

• Alternate foot placement and impact—land sometimes on toes, sometimes heels, sometimes flat footed, heel-toe or toe-heel.

• Alternate jumping/hopping/leaping activities with walking and emphasize correct walking technique (heelstrike on outer edge of heel, roll foot forward, push off with ball of toes, and extend ankle fully).

MINIMIZES REPETITIVE MOVEMENTS

■ When we evaluate instructors, we can usually tell the instructor's "signature" move or series of movements because the move appears over and over again in their warm up or aerobic segment. The most popular "signature moves" are the knee lift and straight leg kicks. Some signature moves are a series of movements from popular dances or routines you've practiced in cheerleading, marching band, or pom-pom squad that are now a part of you. There is nothing wrong with having a "signature move" or "signature series"; however, if this movement or movement pattern is used often at one time (i.e., 50 can-can kicks), you should develop new patterns. You can decrease your number of repetitive movements by visiting other classes, enrolling in a dance class, or attending a choreography exchange. Have your participants share their favorite moves in order to pick up new ideas and fresh combinations.

If you have created some "new moves," be certain to develop the pattern well enough to enable you to make smooth transitions while giving appropriate cues. New movement patterns can be challenging, but this is what makes aerobic activities fun, exciting and interesting.

MAKES SMOOTH TRANSITIONS

■ Transitions are a very difficult aspect of the class to master. It takes time, practice and anticipation to be good at cuing the next movement. Leading the class through smooth transitions is an important aspect of safety, since people tripping over their own feet or bumping into one another create a hazardous situation.

Once you have mastered anticipatory cuing through both practice and experience, it will be much easier to become an exercise educator. You will be able to smile, laugh and enjoy your class as you are cuing, educating, and really getting into your work outs. We encourage you to practice until you are comfortable. Also give your class time to become comfortable with any new movement pattern you have introduced. We mentioned using some time in the warm-up period for instruction, reinstruction, or practice, but occasionally you may have to stop the flow of the exercise class as well. Below are some suggestions for making transitions easier:

- *Keep new moves or movement patterns simple and uncomplicated.* For example: Walk forward 4, do 4 side leg lifts, Walk back 4. Repeat above combination, but add a 1/4 turn and make a box. Once this pattern is mastered, add on another 8 count, or use different arm patterns.

- *Break complicated choreography into smaller sections.* Teach small sections, then begin adding them together one at a time until the entire movement pattern is learned.

- *Alternate choreography with "free" or unchoreographed moves.* Many people are uncoordinated and awkward with choreography. Since people are in your class to feel good about themselves—if you find a participant who is having difficulty and getting frustrated, help him/her out individually or decrease the choreography.

- *Transitions are always more difficult if you are changing direction.* Arrange your sequence of movements so that you are not changing patterns while changing direction.

- *Balance choreography and "free" movement.* The less choreography you use, the less cuing is necessary. Reducing your choreography will decrease your need to cue and transition from one movement to another will be straightforward and easier. This will give you more time to interact with participants.

PROMOTES INDEPENDENCE/SELF-RESPONSIBILITY

■   The promotion of independence and self-responsibility during an exercise class is one of the most important aspects of your leadership. Whether you are leading an exercise class, supervising a circuit class, or using exercise equipment, you cannot be everywhere or help everyone simultaneously. Each participant in your class is working at a different fitness level and for different reasons. If they exercise at your level or another person's level, they may work too hard and sustain an injury or they may not work hard enough. It is important that you constantly encourage everyone by saying "work at your own pace, within your target heart rate range or at the somewhat hard level on the scale of perceived exertion." (Target heart rates and perceived exertion will be discussed in detail in Chapter 6).

Demonstrate high/medium/low intensity moves and teach your class at various levels. Help people achieve the level of effort THEY need to reach their personal targets by teaching them how to modify and monitor their own levels of intensity. You might point out participants in your class who always work at the low intensity level or who modify movements well or who work at higher levels. An excellent instructor will maintain a medium intensity most of the time, but will also present other options and intensities as the need arises.

One of the reasons exercise is a powerful force in people's lives is that they realize to be an "exerciser" requires power, mastery, and choice. Promoting independence and self-responsibility is one of the differences between the performance instructor and the performance educator.

If you are injured, you, too, must demonstrate independence and self-responsibility. Now **you** need to modify your own intensity. If you usually work out during the exercise class, plan to introduce activities that do not require constant demonstration and leadership. This is an opportune time to circulate, correct form, and give encouragement.

PROMOTES PARTICIPANT INTERACTION

■ Along with power, mastery, and choice, people like to exercise in a group setting because they enjoy interacting with other people. You must promote participant interaction in your classes so that participants will get to know each other and reap the social benefits of exercise. Many of our participants derive a great deal of satisfaction and a feeling of belonging from interacting with other class members. This increase in self-esteem, through exercise and social contact, is as important as the physical changes that are taking place.

Here are some suggestions that you might use to increase interaction in your classes:

* Talk to people often, always using names.
* Introduce new people to other members of the class.
* Have people choose partners during the aerobic segment, do hand slaps and have people introduce themselves.
* Keep records of birthdays. Do as many abdominal curls as the participant's age or sing Happy Birthday!
* Use claps, snaps, yells in your aerobic routines. For example: Slap the thighs two times, clap two times, lift the arms two times and yell "HEY" two times.
* Ask people to lead their favorite move or name a part of the body they would like to exercise.
* Use holidays for musical themes and special activities. Circuits are good to use at this time—just put the exercises on pumpkin cut-outs, valentines, or candy canes.
* Have nutritional goodies at the end of class.
* One instructor we know brings a tennis ball to class, particularly when there is a new participant. During the stretching/ relaxation portion of the class he would roll the ball and whomever it touched had to state their name and something significant about themselves.

Involving your participants in this process lets them feel good toward exercise and your class. This camaraderie makes up for the hard work and realities of exercise. Although techniques like these are challenging and frightening (you never know what will happen), such special events make you an extraordinary instructor and keep people coming back for more. YOU CANNOT BEAT THESE TECHNIQUES FOR MAKING EXERCISE FUN AND MEANINGFUL!

EMPHASIZES FUN AND ENTHUSIASM

■ As an exercise instructor, you MUST LOVE WHAT YOU ARE DOING AND BELIEVE IN ITS VALUE! If you do not believe in yourself and the power of exercise, it will be very difficult for you to project fun and enthusiasm. Instructors who really have a good time and enjoy their work are usually the ones who have the biggest, most consistent and loyal followings.

Some days you will look at a drained or angry group of people and wonder what's going on. By inventing a new gimmick or helping your exercise class use physical activity as a catharsis you can watch the energy level rise, and their joy return.

Ask participants if they are having a good time either by a written survey or through direct questioning. Many participants are very willing to let you know if they enjoy your class. FUN is at the core of the exercise class. If the participants are not having fun, then you need to find out why and change your method of instruction.

GRADUALLY DECREASES IMPACT/INTENSITY TO END AEROBIC SEGMENT

■   The last two songs of the aerobic segment should be less intense, but people should be kept moving to prevent blood from pooling in the lower extremities and to allow the cardio-vascular system to make the transition to more gradual workloads. This is especially impera-tive if some type of floor work will follow the aerobic segment. Use words like "Easy, we're slowing down now, move and relax your arms below the level of your heart." We recommend that the last song played in the aerobic segment be at the tempo appropriate for low impact activity, with light easy movements, while keep-ing the hands below the heart to allow for better blood return and decrease the blood pressure.

Checking the pulse rate before proceed-ing to the floor for stretching and relaxation will let people know whether they have recovered enough to begin floor work (heart rate below 100 beats) or if they need to continue walking for a few minutes. Beginning exercisers will need greater time to cool down because their systems are not as efficient. People hate cooling down—BUT DO NOT LET THEM ESCAPE OR FORGET TO COOL DOWN, especially if they have to leave class early.

We are constantly asked what to do about participants who cannot or will not stay be-cause they do not think it is important or they have something pressing to do. One of the statements you might make at the beginning of every exercise class: "If you have to leave early, please stop the aerobic segment a few minutes sooner and cool down before leaving." Then repeatedly remind class members to abide by your request to cool down.

You might also appeal to the comfort and safety issues associated with cooling down.

Because metabolic waste products get trapped inside the muscle cells, most people experience increased cramping and stiffness if they do not cool down. Cooling down enables waste prod-ucts to disperse and the body to return to rest-ing levels without injury. Most people have difficulty arguing with a request that stresses personal safety and comfort.

QUADS AND CALVES STRETCHED IMMEDIATELY AFTER AEROBIC SEGMENT

■   The best time to increase flexibility is when the muscles are warm, pliable, and fa-tigued; therefore, stretching these two muscle groups immediately after the aerobic segment is recommended. Immediately after exercise the quadriceps and gastrocnemius muscles are in prime condition to be stretched because they have been performing the bulk of the aerobic work. Stretching the thighs and calves imme-diately after the completion of the aerobic seg-ment will also assure that those participants who may exit early before the floor work will have performed some essential stretching.

VERBAL DIRECTIONS CLEAR/ MUSIC VOLUME APPROPRIATE

■   We would like to take this opportunity to reiterate the importance of keeping the volume and tempo of the music appropriate for both your participants and the physical setting. We admit that we usually increase the volume of the music for the aerobic segment because it helps motivate our participants. Furthermore, if equipment is being used, it is necessary to increase the volume to be able to hear anything other than the bass. However, extremely loud music will make instructions difficult to hear, especially for the beginners who rely predominantly on your cuing directions. A loud volume will also make your job more difficult since your voice must rise above the level of the music.

MUSIC TEMPO APPROPRIATE FOR BIOMECHANICAL MOVEMENT

■ Counting the number of beats per minute in a song is the fastest way to know whether it will be appropriate for a certain type of movement. Generally speaking, if you use a song that is greater than 160 beats per minute and you try to provide movement for every beat, you will need to greatly reduce the range of motion of the arms and legs to meet that tempo. If you try large movements through full range of motion, you will not only be out of rhythm (which is very annoying to some individuals), but also risk joint injury.

You need to remind your participants that slower music is MORE difficult yet more beneficial because it allows for a greater range of motion which increases muscle and joint involvement, requires more body control, and thereby intensifies the workload. Fast music (160+ beats per minute) decreases intensity because you are moving in a very small range of motion to keep up with the beat. This makes the movement more isometric, decreases blood flow and increases blood pressure.

Most pre-recorded, pre-mixed tapes that you purchase will range from 140-160 beats per minutes in the aerobic segment. The type of music you choose must be at the tempo that fits the biomechanical movement. If you feel you are moving too fast, you probably are! Slow down or use every other beat and use a full range of motion.

References

1. American College of Sports Medicine. 1990. Position statement on the recommended quantity and quality of exercise for developing and maintaining fitness in healthy adults. *Med Sci Sports Exer.* 22:265-274.
2. *Webster's New Twentieth Century Dictionary.* 1972. Unabridged 2nd edition, The World Publishing Company.
3. Cooper, K. 1977. *The Aerobics Way.* Bantam Books.
4. Foster, C. 1975. Physiological Requirements of Aerobic Dancing. *Research Quarterly, 46-1,* 120-122.
5. Igbanugo, V., and Gutin, B. 1975. The Energy Cost of Aerobic Dancing. *Research Quarterly, 49-3,* 308-316.
6. Eickhoff, J., Thorland, W., and Ansorge, C. 1983. Selected Physiological Effects of Aerobic Dancing Among Adult Women. *J Sports Med, 23,* 273-280.
7. Watterson, V. 1984. The Effects of Aerobic Dance on Cardiovascular Fitness. *Phys Sports Med, 10,* 138-145.
8. Johnson, S., Berg, K., and Latin, R. 1984. The Effect of Training Frequency of Aerobic Dance on Oxygen Uptake, Body Composition and Personality. *J Sports Med, 7,* 156-162.
9. Vetter, W., Helfet, D., Spear, K., and Matthews, L. 1985. Aerobic Dance Injuries. *Phys Sports Med, 13-2,* 114-120.
10. Richie, D., Kelso, S., and Bellucci, P. 1985. Aerobic Dance Injuries: A Retrospective Study of Instructors and Participants. *Phys Sports Med, 13-2,* 105-111.
11. Francis, L., Francis, P., and Welshons-Smith, K. 1985. Aerobic Dance Injuries: A Survey of Instructors. *Phys Sports Med, 13-2,* 105-111.
12. Mutoh, Y., Sawai, S., Takanashi, Y., and Skurko, L. 1988. Aerobic Dance Injuries Among Instructors and Students. *Phys Sports Med, 16-12,* 81-88.
13. Claremont, A., Simowitz, S., Boarman, M., Asbell, A., and Auferoth, A. 1986. The Ability of Instructors to Organize Aerobic Dance Exercise into Effective Cardiovascular Training. *Phys Sports Med, 10,* 89-100.

14. Otto, R., Parker, C., Smith, T., Wygand, J., and Perez, H.1988. The energy cost of low impact and high impact aerobic exercise, (abstract.) *Med Sci Sports Exerc18*, 23.

15. Ricard, M., and Veatch, S. 1990. Comparison of Impact Forces in High- and Low-Impact Aerobic Dance Movements. *Inter J Sport Biomechanics*, 6, 67-77.

16. Francis, L., and Francis, P. 1989. Moderate-Impact Aerobics. *IDEA Today Fitness Magazine*, September.

17. Brown, P., and O'Neill, M. 1990. A Retrospective Survey of the Incidence and Pattern of Aerobics Related Injuries in Victoria, 1987-1988. *Australian J. Science and Medicine in Sport.* 22(3): 77-8.

18. Stanforth, D., et al.1991. The Effect of Bench Height and Rate of Stepping on the Metabolic Cost of Bench Stepping, *Med Sci Sport and Exercise* (abstract) 23:4, S143.

19. Olson, M.s. et al. 1991.Cardiorespiratory Reponses to Aerobic Bench Stepping Exercise in Females, *Med Sci Sport and Exercise* (abstract), 23:4, S27.

20. Blessing, D.L. et al.1991. The Energy Cost of Bench Stepping With and Without One and Two Pound Hand-held Weights, *Med Sci Sport & Exercise,*(abstract) 23:4, S28.

21. Goss, F., et al.1989. Energy Cost of Bench Stepping and Pumping Light Hand-held Weights, in Trained Subjects, *Research Quarterly for Exercise and Sport*, 60:4, 369-72.

22. La Forge, R. 1991.What the Latest Research Has to Say about Step Exercise. *IDEA Today*, 31-35, Sept.

23. Koszuta, L.1989. From Sweats to Swimsuits: Is Water Exercise the Wave of the Future? *Phys Sports Med,17:4*, 203-206, 1989.

24. Evans, B., Cureton, K., and Purvis, J. 1978. Metabolic and Circulatory Responses to Walking and Jogging in Water. *Research Quarterly*, 49, 442-449.

25. DeBenedette V. Are Your Patients Exercising Too Much? *Phys Sports Med, 18-8*, 119-122, 1990.

26.Koplan, J.P., Casperson, C.J., and Powell, K.E. 1989. Physical activity, Physical fitness, and Health: time to act. *J Am Med Assn, 262,* 2437.

If we can change
time and space,
we can change ourselves.
We can find new ways
to communicate,
new words to say,
new topics to pursue.
We can find new ways
to operate,
to invent,
to respond.
If I can change
time and space,
I can change habits too.

Cindy Herbert
Susan Russell
Every Child's Everyday

PULSE RATE(PR) OR
RATE OF PERCEIVED EXERTION (RPE) APPLICATION:

- PR/RPE charts are on site & visible or participants know recommended THR
- PR and/or RPE taken after 6-8 min. of activity
- Turns music off for pulse count
- Peripheral pulses, excluding the carotid pulse, are encouraged
- Participants are kept moving during PR counts
- Ten second PR counts are used
- Assistance given to participants having difficulty or unusual results
- Gives modifications based on PR/RPE results and encourages participants to work at individual levels/abilities
- PR not taken too often

Chapter 6

MONITORING INTENSITY OF WORK:
PULSE RATE OR RATE OF PERCEIVED EXERTION APPLICATION

■ In the previous chapter we repeatedly mentioned the need for maintaining a certain level of intense effort to benefit the heart and lungs. We also presented movement possibilities that would allow for modifications in intensity. In this chapter we will actually use "biofeedback" to determine if a person is working at a level that will optimize his/her workout. For many years, exercisers have been counting their heart rate response to workloads and exercise. Heart rates increase as workloads increase. Therefore, we can use our heart rates very much like the RPM gauge in an automobile to determine the direct effect of the workload or the intensity of work on the engine or heart.

We will be covering both the use of target heart rate and perceived exertion. We do not advocate one method of monitoring over the other, as both have application depending on the type of activities your participants will be performing during their exercise session.

TARGET HEART RATE RANGE

■ Everyone in your exercise class should be given instruction regarding the purpose of monitoring his/her heart rate during exercise. They should know how to obtain a pulse and their own personal heart rate range. Posters with target heart rate ranges, conversion charts, (10 second count to beats per minute) and perceived exertion charts should be available in the exercise area to assist the participant.

There are several formulas for determining target heart rate range. Some require a determination of an individual's VO2 max or MET level before they can be used. Two formulas that are commonly utilized to determine a target heart rate range for exercise are the Basic Formula and the Karvonen Formula, which are outlined in Tables 6-1 and 6-2.

Table 6-1

The Basic Formula

Maximal Heart Rate (220-age)
x .50 to .85
= Target Heart Rate Range

Example: 38-year-old
$$220\text{-age} = 182 \qquad\qquad 182$$
$$\underline{\text{x.50}} \qquad\qquad \underline{\text{x.85}}$$
$$91 \quad \text{to} \quad 154.7$$
=Target Heart Rate Range

Table 6-2

Karvonen's Formula

Maximal Heart Rate (220-age)
- Resting Heart Rate (RHR)
x .50 to .85
+ Resting Heart Rate (RHR)
= Training or Target Heart Rate Range

Example: 38-year-old,
resting heart rate, 70 bpm

220-38 = 182

182	182
-70	-70
112	112
x .50	x .85
56	95.2
+ 70 (RHR)	+70 (RHR)
126 to	**165.2**

= **Target Heart Rate Range**

In the examples given in Tables 6-1 and 6-2, you may notice that there is a big difference in the recommended target heart rate ranges for the same participant. The Basic Formula underestimates the target heart rate for a given metabolic level by about 15% (1). Karvonen's Standard Equation is based on establishing a known maximal heart rate value; however, if a person's maximal heart rate is not known and 220 is substituted, it is possible that the suggested target heart rate would overestimate a person's capability.

A maximal heart rate value is established by pushing the person to perform maximal exercise. Maximal exercise is defined by ACSM Guidelines as the point where the person can no longer continue exercising because of fatigue or symptoms, OR when measured maximal oxygen consumption is achieved, and/or there is no further heart rate acceleration with increases in workload. It is important to note that, most exercise participants are NOT stress tested before they begin an exercise program, even though this is frequently recommended; therefore, most exercise participants DO NOT KNOW their true maximal heart rates. Most exercise charts as well as most exercise instructors use the number 220 (the highest heart rate seen in various research projects) rather than a true maximal rate that has been obtained from an

individual participant during an exercise evaluation. This deduction of a person's age from 220 to derive a predicted maximal heart rate is a commonly accepted practice, even though it can be inaccurate. It is this reason that it becomes important to have a target heart rate range. If the participant's maximal heart rate is lower or higher than the estimated maximal heart rate (220-age), the range should take care of this.

Another possibility for error exists when using Karvonen's Equation to add and subtract the resting heart rate. Normal limits of resting heart rate are accepted as 60 to 100 beats per minute. Given these parameters, if a person's rate is below 60 beats per minute the individual is considered to have bradycardia or a slow heart rate. If a person's heart rate is above 100 beats per minute, the individual is said to have tachycardia or a fast heart rate. The reason for either tachycardia or bradycardia may be as simple as position or thought process or as complicated as cardiac disease or level of cardiac function.

Long distance runners, the epitome of cardiopulmonary fitness, have resting heart rates well below 60 beats per minute because their hearts are very efficient and pump a large quantity of blood with each beat. On the other hand, if a person's resting heart rate is 90 beats per minute, the individual might be excited or worried. However, if this value is repeatedly his/her resting value, it would be safe to say that this individual's cardiovascular system while working within normal limits is not as conditioned or efficient as it could be.

As an example, let's show you what could happen if you apply the Karvonen's Equation to two individuals whose resting heart rates are in the upper and lower ranges of normal.

Joe Whobatz is sedentary and his resting heart rate is 90 beats per minute. Josie Batzwho is a very active individual and her resting heart rate is 65 beats per minute. Joe and Josie are both 45 years old.

You can see a discrepancy in the example on the next page. Common sense dictates that Josie should be the person who can work at a higher target heart rate instead of Joe. Remember, the Karvonen Formula was developed to use with a known, established maximal heart rate. Heart rates   close to either end of the normal limits will result in target heart rates that may be either too high or too low.

Joe, the Unfit		Josie, the Fit
220	Predicted Maximal Heart Rate	220
-45	Age	-45
175	Predicted Age-Adjusted Maximal HR	175
-90	Resting Heart Rate	-65
85		110
x.70	Percentage of Intensity for Exercise	x.70
59.5		77
+90	Resting Heart Rate	+65
149.5		
or 150	Recommended Target Heart Rate	142

We recommend that you use the Basic Formula for beginners and advanced exercisers. Although such an equation usually underestimates the target heart rate by 15%, it is better to be conservative, particularly with a beginning exerciser. When you observe that the person is an advanced exerciser, then you can recalculate the Basic Formula at a high work intensity (from 60-85%). The ideal is to obtain a maximal graded exercise test for all participants, but since this is unlikely, and for most people cost prohibitive, use the Basic Formula for beginners and advanced exercisers. Remember that having a range is important.

The recent monitoring of heart rates for intensity of effort during aerobic dance has been questioned as potentially inaccurate (1). The accuracy issue arises because aerobic dance works so much of the upper body musculature with arms frequently raised above the head. These situations cause an increased sympathetic nerve output, which could falsely increase the heart rate because of a pressure overload rather than the volume overload that occurs with lower extremity exercise. Simply expressed, in an aerobic dance class that emphasizes overhead arm work and uses heart rate to measure intensity, you THINK you are working harder than you actually are; therefore monitoring your heart rate can be inaccurate.

Another method of monitoring intensity that is currently gaining popularity is the Rate of Perceived Exertion Scale developed by G.V. Borg (2). This scale was first utilized during graded exercise testing in an attempt to subjectively quantify people's view of their work in-

tensity. During a graded exercise test, exercisers were asked how hard they thought they were working on a scale of 6-20. People could either choose from a numerical scale or descriptors listed next to the numbers. The exercise evaluation was considered to be maximal or near maximal when the individuals being tested would rate their exertion at "19", "20" or "very, very hard" (3). Target heart rate range would be somewhere between "12-15."

Rating of Perceived Exertion

Original rating	Description
6	very, very light
7	
8	very light
9	
10	
11	fairly light
12	
13	somewhat hard
14	
15	hard
16	
17	very hard
18	
19	very, very hard
20	

You might wonder why subjective rating was necessary when the testers were monitoring heart rates and other cardiovascular parameters. As we have discussed previously in the heart rate sections, the formulas used to calculate maximal heart rates are often only predictions that do not correspond to a person's actual maximal heart rate. Also, many individuals take medications that either elevate or blunt their heart rate response, thus invalidating the use of target heart rates. We like the use of perceived exertion to monitor exercise intensity because it teaches participants to analyze their bodies using internal feedback. Often participants get caught up in a "numbers game" of pulse rates instead of focusing on how they feel during exercise.

The 1990 Position Statement by the American College of Sports Medicine on the appropriate exercise techniques for healthy adults recognizes the use of Perceived Exertion as a "valid method of monitoring intensity of exercise." However, this statement reads "It (referring to Rate of Perceived Exertion or RPE) is generally considered an adjunct to heart rate monitoring of relative exercise intensity, but once the relationship between heart rate and RPE is known, RPE can be used in place of heart rate." The position statement goes on to say that there may be certain segments of the population whose heart rate would be critical to the participant's safety, thereby excluding use of RPE for monitoring exercise intensity. We would like to suggest that you use heart rates for beginning exercisers and later introduce the concept of Rate of Perceived Exertion and its relationship to heart rate. Once the participant is well versed in both methods, he or she can choose to use the method that works best.

RPE is especially applicable when you are dealing with people who need to modify their exercise because of their physical condition. For example, a woman participating in a pregnancy exercise class may only have her heart rate at 110 beats per minute during the aerobic segment, but may rate her work intensity at "15" (hard) or "17" (very hard) due to the fatigue and discomfort she feels from pregnancy. The use of RPE in this setting is certainly a valid and helpful way for her to feel that she is working toward greater health while considering her current condition.

Let's proceed to the Exercise Instructor Evaluation Tool to look at the various ways an exercise instructor can help the exerciser monitor intensity during the aerobic segment.

PULSE RATE AND/OR RPE TAKEN AFTER 6-8 MINUTES OF ACTIVITY

■   When an individual starts exercising, the heart rate begins to increase in response to the greater demand activity places on the cardiovascular system. The heart rate rises briskly at first, then as the body adjusts, the heart rate levels off. Heart rates will remain at this level unless the workload increases or decreases. In response to a new demand, the heart rate will again rise and then level off once the cardiorespiratory system has met that demand. This rise and leveling off of heart rate continues until maximal exercise is reached OR there is another change in demand. If exercisers take their pulse soon after beginning exercise, the rate may be on the rise rather than leveled off. It is with these facts in mind that we suggest that heart rates be taken after at least 6 to 8 minutes of activity. This bypasses warming up and transitional aerobics to measure a heart rate that has leveled off or reached a steady state.

TURN MUSIC OFF FOR PULSE COUNT

■   When music is playing, people often end up counting the musical beats rather than their own internal rhythm. For best results, do not just turn the music down, turn it off.

PERIPHERAL PULSES (EXCLUDING THE CAROTID PULSE) ARE ENCOURAGED

■   There are many sites on the body to monitor pulse. Many are inaccessible or hard to use (pedal pulses in the feet or femoral or popliteal pulses in the leg). Other sites are very easy to reach and use for monitoring a pulse as pictured in Figure 6-1: temporal—in front of the ear; radial—at the base of the thumb in the wrist; brachial—on the inner side of the elbow joint; carotid—on the front of the neck.

We do not recommend use of the carotid artery for pulse taking during exercise. Discouraging the carotid site is difficult because the pulse here is strong and people are familiar with this site through CPR classes. However, we have found that when people hear the rationale and are helped to find other sites they will usually comply with this request.

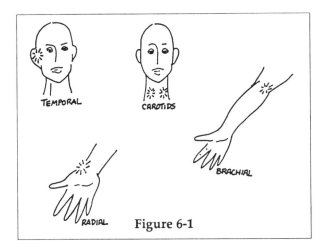

Figure 6-1

The carotid artery bifurcates or splits shortly after passing the clavicle. At this bifurcation in the artery, baroreceptors are found that are very sensitive to pressure. When you press on these baroreceptors, a message is sent to the brain to decrease heart rate and decrease blood pressure because of the lack of oxygen to the brain. Your brain wants you to become horizontal so oxygen can reach the brain quickly. If your participants insist on using the carotid site, not only can they obtain an incorrect reading, but they may also decrease blood flow to the brain.

Medically, carotid sinus massage is used to attempt to change certain cardiac rhythms and decrease rapid heart rates. Even when performed by trained medical personnel, carotid sinus massage (CSM) is a potentially dangerous procedure. In older adults, the CSM procedure has been associated with fainting, stroke, cardiac arrhythmias and stoppage of the heart (4). This increased risk with older people is probably due to the build up of cholesterol plaques in the carotid artery around this region. **Please help your participants find and use alternative sites!**

Two of the best sites are the radial and temporal pulses. Many people have difficulty feeling their pulse here for many reasons—but many of these difficulties can be simply overcome. Try the methods listed below, and see, or rather feel, that they make a difference.

1. Use the flats of the index and middle fingers (not the thumb—it has a prominent pulse of its own). This provides a larger highly sensitive surface area for detecting the pulse.

2. Cock the wrist back (away from the face). This helps to push the artery, which lies deep, closer to the surface.

3. Try to feel the pulse at the base of the thumb. If you cannot locate a pulse here, move the fingers back 1/2" or so and keep trying. Many people find a pulse right where they wear their watchbands. If people are on softer tissue and press, they will diminish or stop the pulse momentarily.

4. PRESS LIGHTLY. When people do not feel a pulse initially, they press harder. They are CORRECT when they say they do not feel anything. They are pressing too hard and cutting off the blood supply.

5. Straighten the arm that is being monitored for pulse. We have found that some people have a diminished pulse when their elbows are bent. Straighten the arm and magically the pulse is intensified and measurable.

6. For beginners, mark the site of the pulse with an "X" or find an anatomical landmark they can use to always locate their pulse.

7. PRACTICE! Many people give up out of embarrassment or frustration. Encourage them to practice often and do not offer to assist them too often or they will expect constant help. Some people do have difficulty because of decreased sensation in their fingertips due to a past injury (frostbite, burns, accidents) or calluses so you may always have to assist some people.

PARTICIPANTS ARE KEPT MOVING DURING PULSE RATE COUNTS

■ If a person is working at high levels and stops suddenly to take a pulse rate count, blood will pool in the lower extremities. It does so because the veins (which pump blood back to the heart) do not work without muscle contraction. As the veins carry blood back to the heart against gravity, they have powerful pumps to assist them. These muscular pumps "shut down" unless muscle contraction comes to their aid. Also, when blood pools in the legs it causes blood pressure to decrease in the head. Spots before the eyes, dizziness, and fainting may result. Therefore, it is important to keep people moving during the pulse rate monitoring:

- Have them walk slowly while counting
- Shift weight from side to side while counting
- Squeeze toes in their shoes
- Step lightly in place

All of these activities require leg movements including lower leg muscle contraction, which in turn keeps the circulation going.

TEN (10) SECOND PULSE RATE COUNTS ARE USED

■   While six second counts are fine and mathematically simple to use (16 for a six-second count x 10 or add a 0 = 160) they can be less accurate than a 10-second count. Since the heart is very efficient, the pulse rate will decrease rapidly in 15 seconds; therefore, the 10-second count is still the best one. Because it is difficult for some people to multiply by 6, be sure to have your conversion charts hanging nearby for easy reference or remind them that what they really need to remember is their 10-second count.

ASSISTANCE GIVEN TO PARTICIPANTS HAVING DIFFICULTY OR UNUSUAL RESULTS

■   As mentioned in previous sections, there are many ways to increase the likelihood of obtaining and counting a correct pulse rate. When someone consistently has trouble, give him or her a little one-on-one instruction or position yourself next to that person before you call a pulse count so you can be available to help. Outlined below are several instances where you may need to check a participant's heart rate yourself:

- If you feel that someone's appearance and breathing rate do not seem to match their reported count.
- If a participant repeatedly reports outrageous counts (either too high or too low).
- If a person reports difficulty because of "skips," "pauses" or "irregular beats."

Sometimes when people are breathing very fast and hard—each time they take a breath there might be a pause in the pulse. Each time the diaphragm contracts for breathing, the major vein (Inferior Vena Cava) that returns from the lower extremity to the heart squeezes shut. This might be the reason for the pause; however, if you cannot synchronize this pause with breathing, the person might be having changes in their heart rhythm and they need to get that checked with a physician before returning to exercise class. Many people have arrhythmias or disarrhythmias of the heart when they are under stress, have had too much caffeine, or are very fatigued—so the problem may not be serious, but it does warrant closer examination by a doctor.

GIVES MODIFICATIONS BASED ON PR/RPE RESULTS AND ENCOURAGES PARTICIPANTS TO WORK AT INDIVIDUAL LEVELS/ABILITIES

■ We believe that each participant should know his/her own target heart rate range. It is your responsibility to provide them with a recommended aerobic target heart rate, instructions on how to use PR or RPE's and then provide opportunities to use them.

We have evaluated instructors who follow all the correct procedures for taking pulse rates but don't modify or apply the results. It is essential that once the PR/RPE has been measured, you instruct participants on what to do if they are above or below what is recommended. Therefore, after the pulse rate count or RPE determination, keep people moving, ask people for their results, and continue with instructions. Listed below are examples of appropriate instructions for modification:

• "If you were below your target, you need to work harder. Use your arms AND legs, increase the size and quality of your movements."

• "If you were right on target—GOOD WORK! Keep it up during the next song or lap."

• "If you were higher than your target, you need to slow down, decrease the range of your arm and leg motions, or keep your movements smooth and light. You don't need to work so hard—see if you can work easier in the next set."

• You can use basically the same verbage for the RPE Scale: If you were rating your work level below 13 —work harder by. . . if you are right at 13—good job. . . if you are higher than 13, and so on. You notice in our examples that not only should you mention modification, you need to state ways of accomplishing that modification.

PULSE RATES NOT TAKEN TOO OFTEN

■ Many instructors like to use their pulse rate counts to take a break from the action. This is fine as long as it is not done three to four times per class. Beginners are the exception. Since they are learning how their bodies react during exercise as well as how to modify activity to reach and stay in their target heart rate zone, taking the pulse rate often is acceptable.

We recommended previously taking a pulse rate after at least 6-8 minutes of activity, but you can also take a pulse rate after finishing an especially difficult song in the aerobic segment, using a piece of equipment, or completing a circuit. Taking the pulse rate before going from aerobic activity to floor work is also a good practice. This will allow those participants whose heart rates are higher than 100 beats per minute to continue cooling down before changing levels. Once again YOU are helping hearts make easier transitions.

Whatever you do, do NOT use the pulse or RPE check as a time to "catch your breath." As soon as the PR or RPE check is over, begin activity again while you give modifications and continue exercising.

References

1. American College of Sports Medicine Guidelines for Exercise Testing and Prescription. 1991. Fourth edition. Philadelphia: Lea & Febiger.
2. Borg, G.A.V. Psychological Bases of Physical Exertion. 1982. *Med Sci Sports and Exer, 14-5*, 377-381.
3. American College of Sports Medicine Position Stand on the Recommended Quantity and Quality of Exercise for Developing and Maintaining Cardiorespiratory and Muscular Fitness in Healthy Adults, 1990, pp. 265-273.
4. Grauer, K., and C. Daniel. 1987. *ACLS: Certification Preparation and A Comprehensive Review*, St. Louis: The C.V. Mosby Company.

■ SEARCH EXERCISE ANALYSIS TOOL

DETERMINE IF THE OVERALL PURPOSE OF THE EXERCISE IS TO IMPROVE FLEXIBILITY OR MUSCLE STRENGTH AND ENDURANCE.

Complete the section below, checking the appropriate boxes under "Yes," "Maybe," or "No."

FLEXIBILITY	Yes	Maybe	No
A. Is it important to perform this exercise to counteract the effects of activities of daily life, work, and/or to prepare for recreational pursuits?	( )	( )	( )
B. Is the exercise shown and cued in a biomechanically correct way, with possible modifications presented?	( )	( )	( )
C. Is there adequate base of support?	( )	( )	( )
D. Does the stretch allow for maximum muscle relaxation and minimization of gravitational pull?	( )	( )	( )
E. Is this exercise performed using controlled, non-ballistic movements?	( )	( )	( )
F. Can this exercise be performed *without* compromising other body parts?	( )	( )	( )

MUSCLE STRENGTH AND ENDURANCE	Yes	Maybe	No
A. Is it important to perform this exercise to counteract the effects of activities of daily life, work, and/or to prepare for recreational pursuits?	( )	( )	( )
B. Is the exercise shown and cued in a biomechanically correct way, with possible modifications presented?	( )	( )	( )
C. Is there adequate base of support?	( )	( )	( )
D. Does the exercise work the muscle(s) through the full and correct joint range of motion?	( )	( )	( )
E. Is this exercise performed using controlled, non-ballistic movements?	( )	( )	( )
F. Can this exercise be performed *without* compromising other body parts?	( )	( )	( )

Chapter 7

SEARCH FOR EXERCISE CHOICES

■ One of the major philosophical differences between our beliefs and those of other exercise educators is that we believe every exercise was created for a reason. Rather than throw out an exercise because it is "not safe," we prefer to analyze it to see whether it is biomechanically correct and appropriate for our participants. If it is incorrect, we try to modify the exercise so it can be used in our classes.

From our experience, most often individuals show up for a particular exercise class because that class fits an available time slot in their daily schedule, not because of the designated class level or content. We also realize that almost all of our teaching has been and remains what we call a "mixed group format."

We developed SEARCH so that YOU could select safe, effective exercises that meet the needs of your participants and give consistency to your exercise classes. The next time you review an exercise video or see an exercise in a class or magazine, you may wonder if a specific move would be effective in your class. Rather than guess if it will work or try it with disastrous results, you can try using this SEARCH exercise analysis tool. While SEARCH deals with stretching and strengthening exercises, the analysis process contains a method of looking at all exercise in a more matter of fact way. Although the SEARCH tool does not address exercises used during the aerobic segment, we know that a certain amount of stretching and strengthening is essential preparation before aerobic activity. Most of you, in order to optimize class time for your participants, provide these activities within the framework of your exercise classes. We would like to introduce the components of SEARCH to get you into an analytical mode. On the opposite page, you will find a complete outline of the SEARCH exercise analysis tool. We will be reviewing this in detail beginning with defining the purpose of an exercise.

DETERMINE IF THE OVERALL PURPOSE OF THE EXERCISE IS FLEXIBILITY OR MUSCLE STRENGTH AND ENDURANCE

■ Do we wish to warm up, stretch, strengthen, cool down or "entertain?" We include the word "entertain" to remind you that every move does not need to have a physiological or biomechanically correct basis. We have viewed many classes that are extremely safe and effective but they are BORING. You must always remember that one of the main reasons participants come to your class is because it is "FUN!" Pictured on the next page is a standing lateral side bend which is an example of a possible "entertainment" move.

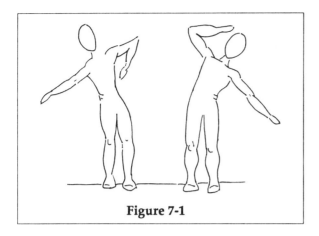

Figure 7-1

This particular move (Figure 7-1) is not a very effective method of strengthening the oblique muscles because there is little added resistance. However, many people enjoy it. We can put this move into our warm up where effectiveness is not our main purpose, but fun, entertainment, and warming up are important. Other examples of "entertainment" moves would be arm swings, finger snapping and clapping. If you cannot decide the purpose of an exercise, you either need to analyze what you are trying to accomplish and why, or perhaps the move can be categorized as an "entertainment" move. As long as the entertainment move follows correct range of motion, avoids jerky/ballistic movements, or is obviously not dangerous, it can be used during the warm up or transitional aerobic phases of a class.

FLEXIBILITY OR MUSCLE STRENGTHENING AND ENDURANCE

■   This section considers six different aspects of any exercise you choose. Each aspect or item can be answered in one of three ways. The scoring is as follows: You may answer questions A through F with "YES," "MAYBE," because the exercise meets some, but not all of the criteria, or you could answer the question with a solid "NO." Check the appropriate box at the end of each question.

An exercise that has six YES scores has met all of the safety criteria and would be good

for everyone, including injured participants. Study any of the MAYBE scores to evaluate what portions of the exercise could be modified to meet the six criteria. Thinking through the modifications will help you determine any cuing that you might need to modify the exercise for individual variations. Consider any of the NO responses for modification as well. A NO SCORE THAT CANNOT BE MODIFIED NEEDS FURTHER ANALYSIS. Is this exercise really necessary? Does the risk outweigh the benefit? An exercise that has components that cannot be modified should be used with extreme caution and only with selected groups or individuals. Other factors to consider are frequency of use and duration of the particular exercise. These aspects need to be considered before using this exercise in a class situation. Cuing, alternatives, and demonstration also need to be prepared.

The purpose of this type of analysis is to get you to consider more carefully the effectiveness, safety, and purpose of an exercise. Let's review the point-by-point analysis A-F of the SEARCH exercise analysis tool in more detail.

■   *Item A: Is it important to perform this exercise to counteract the effects of daily living, work and/or to prepare for recreational pursuits?*

This is a loaded question demanding a great deal of consideration. It also requires knowledge of your class participants and/or that you consider the importance of maintaining muscle balance and ratios because you teach a mixed format.

Let's take a moment to review which muscles need stretching and strengthening in our daily lives. Generally speaking (we will be more specific later), it is the extensor muscles that need to be strengthened for muscular endurance. Major extensor muscles include triceps, hamstrings/gluts, and lower back. The upper back and shins are not extensor muscles but need to be included in the "to strengthen" group. These muscles tend NOT to be used in daily activities and are made weaker by poor posture and sitting. They are often used as stabilizers or postural muscles. Static positioning (holding or maintaining a position over a period of time) also takes its toll. The flexor muscles are used more in our daily activities because we need them to walk forward and perform work in front of us. These muscles need to be stretched. Flexor muscles include biceps, quadriceps, calves and hip flexors.

Remember that this is a basic overview for all participants. If you know their needs, you can meet them more effectively. For example, if you teach the 5:30 p.m. class in downtown Chicago, many of your participants may work at a desk from 8 a.m.-5 p.m. Concentrating on strengthening the abdominals, upper and lower back muscles and stretching the hamstrings, hip flexors and chest/shoulder muscles in EVERY class is appropriate. This regimen will help improve posture and increase the muscular endurance necessary to maintain the static positioning required by their jobs without creating additional stress.

Many of our participants are also active in recreational sports. We can promote the concept that exercise will help someone prepare for their sport, thereby decreasing injury. When softball season is starting, increase your shoulder stretching and strengthening exercises. For golf, practice swings, pivots, and trunk rotation. For basketball and volleyball, add jumping activities. For skiers, practice the moguls by strengthening the thighs and working on balance. Prepare your people before they hit the courts, fields, and slopes. They will thank you many times over for your prior planning to make their recreational pursuits more enjoyable.

Many recreational activities and sports take a toll on the human body. Sports were not developed around human capabilities, but rather as a challenge to human performance. Most recreational activities are shaped by the traditions and ideas handed down from professional sports. But unlike professional athletes, your participants often have sore muscles for days after a recreational activity.

Many individuals still try to use sports to get into shape when they already should have been at a high fitness level. In professional sports, the days of showing up at training camp fat, sassy, and out of shape no longer exist. You not only assist people in maintaining their fit-

ness levels so they can participate, but your class may also be the place where "weekend athletes" and "wounded warriors" return for rebuilding and rehabilitation.

You might be able to help your participants counteract the effects of their recreational and sports activities with gentle stretching, strengthening, and endurance activities. However, you need to know which exercises are safe and effective so that you do not aggravate any further damage. You may also need to refer your participants to physical therapists, sports medicine and rehabilitation physicians, athletic trainers, exercise physiologists and others to get the help they need. Your participants may actually come to you for permission to do what they know they should have already done—get medical treatment as quickly as possible.

We believe it is important that exercise educators strive to develop our participants' understanding of what exercise can do. We want participants to leave our classes feeling better. We want them to take the benefits of our exercise session somewhere beyond the exercise class and into their daily living, which is why Item A is one of the most important questions we need to ask in analyzing an exercise.

■ *Item B: Is the exercise shown and cued in a biomechanically correct way with possible modifications presented?*

Chapter 8 will describe in detail the biomechanics of each major muscle group and discuss tips for cuing and modification. It is essential that you understand how the body moves in order for your participants to have an effective and safe workout.

■ *Item C: Is there an adequate base of support?*

In mixed groups or in a class where there is an injured participant, many of your modifications will consider the base of support first. What we mean by adequate base of support is that when performing an individual stretching or strengthening exercise you feel "stable." Let's look at an example: Figure 7-2 is an exercise many of us use in our classes.

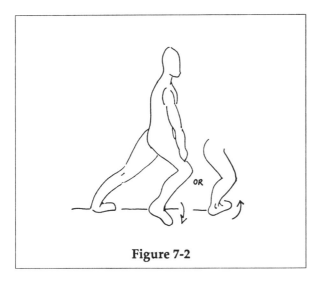

Figure 7-2

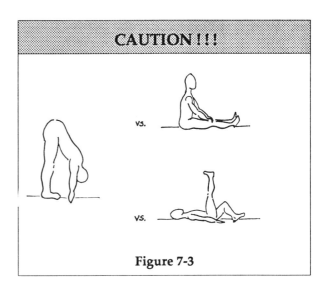

Figure 7-3

This particular calf stretch can be a bit unstable, especially for beginning exercisers. When both toes are pointed directly forward, it can be difficult to maintain balance. The back toe NEEDS to be pointing forward for biomechanical effectiveness; however, the front toe can be turned in or out slightly to make a better base of support and thus provide participants with a more comfortable exercise that is still effective. Placing the hands against the wall or on the back of a chair also increases the base of support, and therefore, stability.

Items D and E deal separately with stretching and strengthening/endurance exercises because each have different components to be assessed.

■   *Item D for stretching: Does the stretch allow for maximum muscle relaxation and minimization of gravitational pull?*

Stretching is more effective when a muscle is relaxed. Therefore, standing stretches are not as effective for leg muscles. A standing bent over hamstring stretch (Figure 7-3) eccentrically contracts the hamstring muscles to save us from falling forward.

In the standing position, the hamstrings are contracting against the gravitational pull of the earth. We will always be working against the effects of the earth's gravity, so seated or lying leg stretches are more effective for increasing flexibility because they minimize this force.

■   *Item D for strengthening: Does the exercise work the muscle(s) through the full and correct joint range of motion?*

The figures on the next page summarize joint range of motion, which will be discussed in further detail in Chapter 8. A point to keep in mind is that range of motion norms are based on averages for groups of people. The degree of an individual's range of motion depends on our genetic make-up and exercise routine. There are also times when working the muscle through the full and correct range of motion is not emphasized. Furthermore, there are situations when moving a joint through the full range of motion, whether by force, increased repetitions, or additional load (weight), could seriously injure that joint. For example, the shoulder capsule, particularly the rotator cuff, could be permanently injured by using a weightlifting machine that forces the participant into an extreme range before the lift (i.e., Nautilus chest or pullover machine, or other types of military press). Shoulder injury could also occur during a fast-paced aerobics class with extreme swinging of the arms or repeated full range movements, particularly if done with hand weights. With these exceptions, particularly during floor work, we still recommend using the full range of motion unless otherwise indicated.

■ JOINT RANGE OF MOTION

HIP AND KNEES

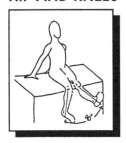

Knee extension: 90°

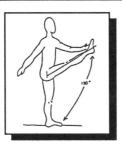

Hip flexion: 120°

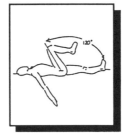

Hip flexion with knee flexion: 120°

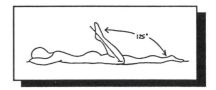

Knee flexion: 125°

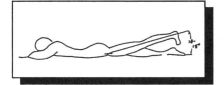

Hip hyperextension: 10 - 15°

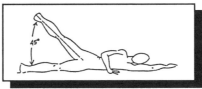

Hip abduction: 45°

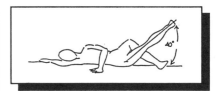

Hip adduction: 40°

SPINE

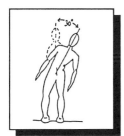

Spinal lateral bending: 30°

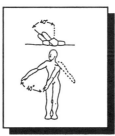

Spinal rotation: 40°

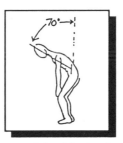

Spinal flexion/ standing: 70°

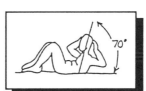

Spinal flexion/lying down: 70°

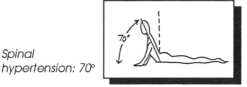

Spinal hypertension: 70°

ARMS/SHOULDER

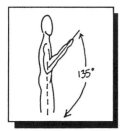

Arm flexion: 135°

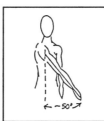

Shoulder adduction: 50°

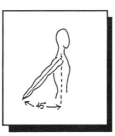

Shoulder hyperextension: 45°

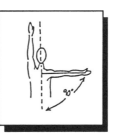

Shoulder abduction: 90-180°

NECK

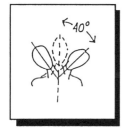

Abduction and Adduction: 40°

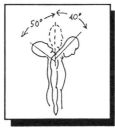

Hyperextension: 50° Flexion: 40°

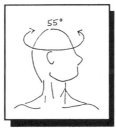

Rotation: 55°

FOOT

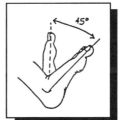

Plantar flexion of foot: 45°

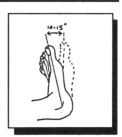

Dorsi flexion of foot: 10-15°

■   *Item E for stretching: Is this exercise performed using controlled, non-ballistic movements?*

Item E for strengthening: Is this exercise performed using controlled, isotonic, non-ballistic movements?

Our concern here is that uncontrolled, ballistic (jerky or pulsing) movements may result in injury to muscle, tendon, and ligamentous tissues. Many people still bounce while stretching and perform strengthening exercises (with or without equipment) as quickly and as forcefully as possible. During aerobic exercise, particularly with fast music tempos, movements often become shortened, more isometric, and ballistic, thus leading to changes in blood flow and blood pressure as well as the possibility for musculoligamentous injury. There is still controversy over whether an isometric muscle contraction is a safe form of muscle strengthening. Outlined below are the basic differences between an isometric muscle contraction and an isotonic muscle contraction (1).

Differences Between Isometric and Isotonic Muscle Contractions

Isometric

A.   A contraction that occurs against an *immovable* object. An example of an isometric exercise would be pushing against a wall.
B.   There is little or no blood flow occurring in the muscle, which may result in a rapid increase in blood pressure and muscular pain because the muscle is"screaming for oxygen."
C.   Strength can be developed using isometric contractions, but it is difficult to measure how much strength is gained.
D.   Strength is not developed through the total range of motion of a joint.

Isotonic

A.   The muscle shortens and there is movement of a limb. An example of an isotonic exercise is a bicep curl.
B.   Blood flow to the muscle is rhythmic and pumps blood in with every movement, therefore, intramuscular tension remains constant.
C.   Strength can be developed utilizing low repetition/high resistance, or muscular endurance can be developed utilizing high repetition (10 or more) and low resistance. Progress can be monitored by increasing weight or repetitions resulting in greater motivation and compliance.
D.   Strength/endurance is developed through a greater range of motion.

Although isometric muscle contractions do increase the strength of the muscles, there are risks to performing an isometric exercise, especially by participants with cardiovascular compromise (high blood pressure, high cholesterol levels, smokers, history of heart disease or stroke).

We will describe an isotonic muscle contraction in more detail as we define the "shortening" and the "lengthening" phase of such a muscle contraction.

The "shortening" phase is called a **concentric** muscle contraction. During this type of contraction, the muscle shortens as it develops tension and overcomes resistance. Examples of a concentric muscle contraction are:

•   the hamstrings group when flexing the knee
•   the bicep group when flexing the lower arm to the shoulder.

The "lengthening" phase of the movements described above would be defined as an **eccentric** muscle contraction and are as follows:

- the hamstring group when extending the knee
- the bicep group when extending the lower arm to waist.

When a muscle contracts eccentrically, the resistance overcomes the active muscle and the muscle lengthens while developing tension. This usually occurs as a muscle acts to oppose the force of gravity (2). It is important to be familiar with muscle contraction terminology. We will be using these terms in Chapter 8 when we are discussing specific exercises and how they affect body parts.

■ *Item F: Can the exercise be performed WITHOUT compromising other body parts?*

In order to provide variety an exercise instructor will often select an exercise that may seriously compromise other body parts. An example is the yoga plough pictured below.

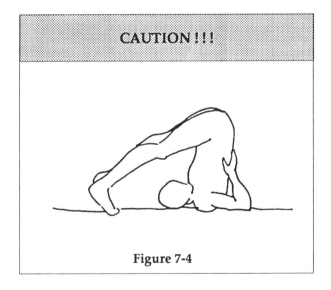

CAUTION !!!

Figure 7-4

This can be an effective stretch for the hamstrings/low back area; however, most of the body's weight is placed on the cervical spine. This could potentially cause neck pain or severe injury. (In Chapter 9 this example will be analyzed with modifications presented.) The risks of this exercise far outweigh the benefits. Other less compromising exercises could be selected to stretch the hamstrings and low back.

The yoga plough is an excellent example of movement selected from a different system of exercise. Yoga, like the martial arts (karate, kung fu, judo), follows a very stringent, highly supervised, and slow progression. Participants perform many movements and activities that prepare them to do the extreme positioning illustrated above. It is important to note that they do not start out with this exercise. While we encourage education and participation in these activities and possible inclusion of some of the techniques, movements and exercises in a class for the general public, it is still essential to be able to eliminate and modify dangerous exercises and positioning.

In summarizing the SEARCH exercise analysis tool, it is important to remember that after going through the point-by-point analysis we need to study questions that were answered "No" or "Maybe." Look at the aspects of the exercise that might be changed, to make the exercise better or to decrease its risk and increase its benefit. We will be using this analysis tool throughout this book. SEARCH is at the heart of our exercise beliefs and practices. Now that you have read this chapter, you can see how SEARCH helped us structure information in Chapter 1, and why we emphasize the important responsibility you have as an exercise instructor—from knowing your participants and making the exercise environment safe to your personal appearance and style. Hopefully this chapter has clearly expressed our belief that all exercisers should be taught by an educator/ performer who understands the importance of optimum safety, educational opportunities, and positive environments, and provides these in her or his class.

References

1. McArdle, W., Katch, F., and Katch, V. 1986. *Exercise Physiology, Energy, Nutrition, and Human Performance.* Philadelphia: Lea and Febiger.
2. Howley, E., and Franks, B. 1986. *Health/ Fitness Instructor's Handbook.* Champaign, IL: Human Kinetics.

"If you should tell me once,
and for some reason I do not understand you,
tell me that I did not listen
and I'll doubt that you can teach me.

If you should tell me once
and for some reason I do not understand you,
tell me that perhaps you did not explain it well—
and I'll know that you can teach me."
—Rosalie Bryant

MUSCULAR STRENGTH/ENDURANCE/ STRETCHING:

- Verbal cues on posture/alignment
- Encourages and demonstrates good body mechanics
- Instructs/encourages breathing technique
- Observes participants' form and suggests adaptations for injuries/special needs
- Corrects/recommends changes in polite, non-threatening way
- Equipment is used safely/effectively (weights, rubber bands, etc.)
- Verbal directions clear/music volume is appropriate
- Music tempo appropriate for biomechanical movement

POST STRETCH/RELAXATION

- Relaxation/energize is emphasized appropriately

FLOOR WORK/ MUSCLE GROUP/ JOINT STRUCTURE REVIEW

The introduction to the SEARCH exercise analysis tool was designed to get you to see the complexity of choosing exercises for your class. In this chapter on muscular strength, endurance, and flexibility we will be sharing with you many exercises we have reviewed. Before we get into the actual exercises, we thought it would be a good time to discuss some general principles of stretching and strengthening.

PROMOTING MUSCLE BALANCE

■   Muscle imbalance is often the cause of an injury to muscles, tendons, and/or ligaments. Any gains made through exercise will be diminished by an injury and overall mental and physical health will be compromised. Therefore, teaching exercise with consideration for what muscles and other structures can and cannot do is essential. Furthermore, consideration of what musculoligamentous structures are often forced to do during daily, work, and recreational activities is at the center of all muscle strengthening and stretching instruction.

The first step in promoting muscle balance is to go back to the participants' health history forms to review what activities your participants perform daily.

Most muscle imbalances arise from lack of muscular balance in our daily activities, so keep in mind what your students do when they are *not* in an exercise class. Then, analyze which muscle groups your students need to develop to counterbalance the muscles they primarily use in daily activities. Concentrate your energy and instruction on the development of opposing muscle groups, to those used daily.

Keep in mind that when we are discussing muscle balance we are not necessarily talking about a one-to-one (1:1) balance. There is *relative* balance between muscle groups that keeps them functioning correctly. For example, the quadriceps muscles are bigger and stronger than the hamstring muscles because we walk forward most of the time. The quadriceps group is two times stronger than the hamstring group, or in other words, the ratio of quadriceps to hamstrings is two-to-one (2:1).

If most work in your exercise class emphasizes strengthening the quadriceps group, the ratio may increase from 2:1 to 3:1 or 4:1, which will result in increased potential for injury to the hamstrings, since they will not have the strength to oppose or stabilize the quadriceps and the knees during exercise and other activities. Therefore, your exercise instruction needs to focus on developing the hamstring muscle groups rather than the quadriceps group. To achieve this you might have to reformat your class to:

- include two to three hamstring strengthening and stretching exercises
- exclude quadriceps strengthening.

Of course, what you do will depend on the needs of your participants and what type of class you are teaching. If you are teaching a mixed group, as most of us do, we encourage you to lead your classes so that muscles that are shortened during our activities of daily living are stretched during the exercise session, and muscles that are stretched daily are strengthened. In order to do this, you need to know opposing muscle groups, how they move reciprocally, or in opposition.

Some examples of opposing or reciprocal muscle groups are:

Opposing Muscle Groups	
Quadriceps	Hamstrings
Abdominals	Spinal Extensors
Pectorals	Rhomboids/Trapezius
Biceps	Triceps
Deltoids	Latissimus Dorsi
Gastrocnemius	Tibialis Anterior
Abductors	Adductors

Notice that the muscle groups in the left hand column are predominantly muscles that are in the front of the body. These muscles become shortened because they are used more often in daily activities. As humans, we have a frontal orientation. In other words, we walk forward, and have our eyes set in the front of our heads, which leads us to perform most activities in front of us. This forward orientation often leads to overdevelopment of the musculature on the front of the body, and weakening of the musculature on the back of the body.

Generally we recommend that you emphasize *strengthening* the muscles in the right hand column, and *stretching* the muscles in the left hand column. Although you may have participants that need a deviation from this scheme, we use this concept as the foundation for our overall class content. There are no hard and fast rules regarding the relative balance of some muscle pairs, notably the abductors and adductors, and the abdominals and spinal extensors. Their balance depends on an individual's posture and how he or she moves in daily activities, so you may find different viewpoints regarding stretching and strengthening these muscle pairs.

You should note that some muscle groups cross more than one joint structure, and therefore the movements are more complex than just flexion or extension. For example, the muscles of the hamstring group originate from the pelvis and attach below the knee joint; therefore, the hamstring group is responsible for both *extending* the hip and *flexing* the knee. Both of these actions need to be included when strengthening the hamstrings.

Other opposing muscle groups that perform reciprocally, are the gastrocnemius muscle (calf) and the anterior tibialis (shin). The gastrocnemius muscle is responsible for plantarflexing the foot (pointing the toe), while the anterior tibialis is responsible for dorsiflexing the foot (pulling the foot toward the face, as on the heelstrike of walking). Since we walk forward and use our calves to jump, we plantarflex more, so we should strengthen the tibialis anterior. For brisk walking classes the opposite is true, since the shins are worked to a greater degree.

Sometimes it is important to look at the function and size of the muscle groups. The deltoid muscles are one of several muscles that oppose the latissimus dorsi. The "lats," as they are commonly called, are huge muscles that sit on either side of the spine and attach to each humerus (upper arm). It is this muscle that when contracted brings the arm down from an overhead position. The deltoid muscles that cap each shoulder are much smaller in mass than the lats. Based on size alone, you might anticipate that we would suggest that you strengthen the deltoids. Rather, we have suggested that the deltoids be stretched and the lats strengthened. Why? Our reasoning has to do with function.

With arms raised overhead, the lats are assisted by gravity in bringing the arms down. The deltoids must lift against gravity to bring the arms into an upward position. During the day, many people must reach repeatedly overhead and in different planes in order to accomplish work tasks. Many exercise instructors unwittingly add to the labor of the deltoid muscles in a flexed position (arms, out to the side, small arm circles, hands forward, hands back) while performing aerobics. It is for these reasons that we include the deltoids in the "to stretch" list.

BALANCING STRENGTH AND FLEXIBILITY

■   Another aspect of balance is the "relative balance" that exists between the strength and the flexibility of a particular muscle group. If the exerciser has a great deal of flexibility in a particular muscle group, you may need to *emphasize strengthening*, rather than flexibility exercises in order to avoid injury to joint structures and ligamentous tissues. If the exerciser has greater strength than flexibility in a particular muscle group, you may need to perform flexibility exercises to avoid strains to the muscles and tendons. We often have the misconception that MORE flexibility and MORE strengthening is beneficial. It is the "relative balance" between flexible *and* strong muscles that create a healthy system.

Ideally you would "assess" each person so that you could recommend the appropriate workout for each. Those of you that are personal trainers and are working with athletes need to set up individual programs that will be most beneficial for each person. Those of you working in a group setting will need to analyze individuals, but present the balance between flexibility and strength to the group as a whole,

and assist individuals in applying the concepts to themselves.

For example, you may have decided to use the sit and reach exercise to stretch the hamstring group, and to measure the hamstring flexibility of your class participants.

The sit and reach exercise is often employed as a field test to screen people for potential low back problems. The assumption is that individuals with tight hamstrings will have a greater risk of back injury since they will be pulled out of correct alignment. The norms used to score the sit and reach test often give an excellent score to those people who can reach the farthest (hands past the feet or palms flat on the wall). This test or information—often given when instructing the sit and reach exercise—is misleading, inaccurate, and ineffective.

Individuals who can touch their toes in a sitting or standing position are often bending at the waist, and not at the hip. Bending at the waist is not an accurate measure of hamstring flexibility, but rather flexibility of the thoracic and lumbar vertebrae. Performing the exercise or test by bending at the hip instead of the waist more accurately assesses the hamstring group. Low back problems are more complex than just having one shortened or stretched muscle group.

Furthermore, use of the sit and reach for an exercise or a test of flexibility can encourage overflexibility by giving an excellent score to those people who can reach the farthest (hands past the feet or palms flat on the wall). The main objective of the sit and reach as an exercise is to stretch the hamstrings, minimizing the effects of gravity. Many people have been injured trying to stttrrreeetttccchhh just a little further.

Also consider that most people should AVOID this position on a daily basis. Bending at the waist without support while working is discouraged. If we include the full sit and reach, ask yourself the question — who <u>works</u> in this position anyway? Our tests and our exercises should always simulate the form and correct technique we want people to use. Why test our exercise participants in a way that continues to reinforce bad habits and unhealthy movement patterns? How do you make this test or exercise work for your participants?

Table 8-1

Sit & Reach Test Revised Norms	
Excellent	Potential risk for injury if not balancing stretching with strengthening exercises.
Good	Maintain current stretching program, but balance with strengthening exercises.
Average	Stretching program is adequate.
Fair	Moderate risk for muscular injury due to inflexible muscles.
Poor	High risk for muscular injury. Begin stretching now.

As a field test for hamstring tightness — give very explicit instruction (i.e., "bend at the hip — NOT the waist; Go to where you can feel the stretch — do not overstretch"). Analyze the highly flexible individuals — Have they had joint injuries or ligamentous injuries? — If so, emphasize the importance of strengthening vs. stretching the hamstring group. Analyze the inflexible individuals — Have they had strains, muscles cramping, trigger points? — Then emphasize the need for stretching vs. strengthening the hamstring group. Outlined in Table 8-1 are the revised norms we use for the sit & reach test.

As an exercise for stretching the hamstring—again give very explicit instructions on how to perform the exercise correctly (i.e., use examples as above and — "Keep your head up—point your chin toward your feet, use your hands to walk your torso forward until you feel the stretch. Use your hands to walk your torso into an upright position, so that you do not use your back to lift."). Format and instruct your class to meet the needs of the participants. If you are working in a group setting this may be difficult to accomplish, but present each exer-

ciser with the opportunity and task of doing what is correct for him/her, then facilitate and prompt him/her as needed.

Another example of the importance of appropriate emphasis on stretching or strengthening can be applied to both the athlete or the normal adult with back problems. Gymnasts, the epitome of flexibility—especially of the spine, have high rates of back pain and injury. Their back pain is associated with overflexible joint structures caused by overstretching of the ligaments of the spine. Strong muscles may be able to compensate for this hyperflexible condition, but if strengthening exercises are eliminated, pain and injury continue to weaken the spinal structure. The extremely flexible nature of the sport of gymnastics means that back and abdominal strengthening exercises are essential to any gymnast's program. After a gymnast leaves the sport, he/she needs to continue these strengthening exercises to maintain adequate function, since the damage done while participating is very likely irreversible and will continue to be a problem.

People that have suffered an injury from an accident, or repetitive motion injuries of the spine, in which the ligaments might be overstretched, also have similar problems. As long as they perform their strengthening exercises, they can control and maintain a reasonable level of pain and/or function. When the individual stops back strengthening exercises, his/her pain increases and re-injury may result. Some individuals can tell immediately that they have decreased function, other people have to wait before they notice increased pain and loss of function. These people, such as ex-gymnasts, need to continue strengthening exercises daily to maintain function and control pain.

In the final analysis, you as the instructor, need to be able to recognize what muscle/muscle group is responsible for a specific action, and what muscle group works in opposition to that action. You need to consider what exercise you will choose to enable your participants to function optimally during exercise and in their daily lives.

PRINCIPLES OF STRENGTHENING

■ Before we begin to discuss the principles of strengthening, we need to define muscle strength and endurance.

Muscle strength is the ability of the muscle(s) to perform maximal work one time only.
For example: How much weight can you lift ONE time?

Muscle endurance is the ability of the muscles to perform the same amount of work or movement repeatedly.
For example: How many curl-ups can you do until you can no longer repeat the movement?

Most exercise instructors include some form of muscle strengthening and endurance in their classes. Some instructors have included this type of exercise as a matter of convention. Others recognized that in order to promote total fitness they had to include exercises for maintaining muscular strength, endurance, and tone, as well as exercises for flexibility and aerobic fitness. Our participants expected this total regime, too!

Recently, the American College of Sports Medicine (ACSM) has included guidelines for resistance/strength training in the 1990 Position Statement on exercise for healthy adults.(1) According to ACSM, most healthy adults need to perform resistance training at least two times per week in order to maintain a minimum level of strength and endurance. ACSM goes on to recommend that each session should include at least one set (8-12 repetitions to "near fatigue") of resistance exercises for all major muscle groups.

If you are teaching mixed groups, we advocate endurance exercises *without* resistance or weight (other than a person's own body weight) until participants are strong enough to lift their own body weight for 20 repetitions or so. Resistance devices should not be utilized until basic strength is acquired. Strength spe-

cialists have indicated that an increase in muscular strength could also be associated with an increase in muscular endurance (1,2,3). As maximal strength increases, the percentage of maximal strength required to lift a given submaximal weight decreases. Therefore, there may be more of a crossover between strength and endurance training than we thought. Watch the developing research carefully for changes in this area.

If your class population already performs many repetitive motions throughout the day (i.e., computer data entry, typing, assembly line or machine work, warehouse and delivery work) they are already at increased risk for repetitive motion injury. Therefore, decrease their risk by limiting the amount of repetitive or endurance movements on hands, wrists, elbows, shoulders, knees, and backs.

For participants who have jobs or activities that require heavy physical demand, emphasize strengthening exercises by using higher weight (lower repetitions), or different resistance other than their own bodies can provide. Sometimes participants who have been in your class *forever* may need a challenge or increased work for special activities (fun runs, recreational sports, etc.). You might add external resistance or weight during floor work. The use of rubber bands, ankle or hand weights, surgical tubing, balls, and other devices will help meet these extraordinary needs. Some individuals may also need to participate in a separate weight training program to meet their needs.

Outlined below are some general principles to keep in mind when organizing the floor work section of your class:

1. *Stress adaptation:* Increasing the intensity of the workout by increasing the number of repetitions, weight, or resistance should be gradual and progressive. Sudden increases in intensity (i.e., doubling the number of repetitions, weight or resistance) could result in muscle damage. Cue and instruct your participants so stress adaptation can occur — "Add one to two pounds if you are able to perform

15 or more repetitions." "Go to the next thickness of rubber band and remember your number of repetitions should be decreased."

2. *Rebuilding time:* When a muscle is stressed beyond its normal limitations, time is needed for repair, recovery, and positive physiological change. Generally, 1-2 days (24 to 48 hours) is required, so resistance and particularly strength training should be performed every other day. Training can occur daily, but different muscle groups need to be emphasized. For example, do strength training for arms and torso on Monday, Wednesday, and Friday; legs on Tuesday and Thursday.

3. *Controlled speed of movement:* Slow, smooth, and controlled movement ensures consistent application of force throughout the range of movement. Keep in mind that faster music tempos (130+ bpm) use more momentum. Slower music tempos (116 bpm) demand control and strength. If you want to progress a class, use slower music tempos as the class session proceeds.

4. *Full range of motion:* Use the full range of motion of the muscle and joint structure to help preserve flexibility. Training the muscles and tendons through a greater range of motion enables more muscle fibers to perform work. "Pulsing" (or performing only a limited range of motion) is discouraged, unless limited range of motion is your goal, as in some abdominal work. Limited range of motion is appropriate for rehabilitation or avoidance of injury, for example: avoiding full range of motion during weight training to avoid injuring the rotator cuff.

5. *Training specificity:* To increase muscle endurance, train with less resistance and more repetitions. If you want to increase muscle strength, emphasize weight/resistance and decrease repetitions. Indi-

viduals who need equal amounts of strength and endurance (triathletes) have a difficult time training to meet and maintain both of these demands.

We often stretch a muscle group immediately after strengthening or endurance work to promote relative balance between flexibility and strengthening a particular group of muscles. Coupling a strengthening/endurance exercise with stretching helps make certain you have included both aspects in your class format, and promotes the optimal benefit of each.

The following includes some examples of cuing that we use in our classes during the stretching and strengthening segments to optimize the educational opportunities.

GENERAL CUING FOR STRENGTHENING EXERCISES

- "Perform this exercise slowly, smoothly, and with control."
- "Breathe in, and as you begin the movement, perform the work, lift the weight, or pull against the resistance -EXHALE!"
- "The number of repetitions is not as important as *tuning in* to the area you are working. When you feel increased warmth, tingling, tightness, —STOP!"
- "Isolate and work only this muscle group, relax all other muscle groups."
- "Correct form is more important than number of reps or amount of weight!"
- "You can do one side until fatigued; then switch to the other side or alternate sides each time."
- "If you are a beginner, stop when you get tired, or change sides even though the rest of the class keeps going."
- "We are going to strengthen the outer thigh through the full range of motion, which is 45°."
- "Even though we are doing many repetitions, this type of exercise will NOT remove fat from this area. To remove fat you need aerobic exercise. This exercise

WILL help you tone and shape muscles and allow you to tuck in, pull up, and contour your body."

In Chapter 4 we discussed the stretch reflex and other principles important to safe and effective stretching. Refer back to Chapter 4 if you need to review the detailed information on stretching.

GENERAL CUING FOR STRETCHING EXERCISES

- "Stretching should be *comfortable*. It should not hurt or cause pain!"
- "Stretching during rehabilitation may be *uncomfortable* but should not increase pain!"
- "During this stretch you may not feel anything but comfort—That's okay! You are maintaining flexibility and preventing injury!"
- "Avoid bouncing or overstretching. Either of these will shorten or contract the muscles. Shortened muscles cannot be stretched, so you are defeating your purpose and risking injury!"
- "Stretch to the point of tension; then hold the stretch and relax."
- "Listen to your body. Listen for comfort, relaxation, easy stretching."
- "Your goal is not to touch your foot, but rather to keep your knee straight in order to stretch optimally."
- "Check your position—Are your toes straight ahead? Is your knee straight? Is your leg straight out in front of you?"
- "Hold each stretch for 10-20 seconds during warm ups, and 20-30 seconds for increasing flexibility *or* if you do not like counting, take 3-4 deep breaths while holding each stretch."
- "Position yourself so that you can achieve maximum muscle relaxation and minimize the effects of gravity during the stretch."

- "At any time during the exercise period or during any activity, if a muscle is tight, *stop and stretch!*"

Once again you can see that you *must* know the exercise goals of your participants to be able to assist them to reach their objectives. They need to know the rationale behind your training methods. It is also important that you emphasize self-responsibility and teach in such a way that your participants are able to accomplish their goals safely and effectively.

Now that you have an idea of the basic principles of stretching and strengthening exercises, we will look at each major muscle group in detail. We will review the names of the major muscles, their actions, and joint ranges of motion. We will then proceed with specific exercises for each muscle group that need to be viewed with caution, and continue with recommended exercises. The exercises presented under each "caution" heading will be addressed in detail. Under the "recommended" exercises, we will present pictures and actual cuing/phrases to encourage participants to strengthen or stretch effectively. *Please do not consider the caution/recommended exercises as do's or don't's!!* This is not the intended purpose.

For years we refused to label exercises with "caution" or "recommended" since many people seeking the cookbook approach will go no further to analyze or adapt, but just take our word as gospel. We have been forced to compromise, since many instructors feel that those labels — as well as pictures and discussion — actually help them understand and analyze more effectively.

Please be advised that the labels "caution" and "recommended" refer to teaching a mixed group with varied goals, fitness levels, and personal needs. Many of these caution and recommended exercises may need to be adapted or modified to meet the needs of special populations (obese, pregnant, pulmonary patients, elderly, injured, or arthritic to name a few).

Our goal is to select exercises that will improve the health and quality of life for our particular class population(s). We cannot be certain that specific exercises are harmful to everyone or anyone in particular(4), although based on individual trial and error, and an accumulation of anecdotal evidence, we do know what affects many individuals. Scientific data linking specific injuries to a particular exercise is certainly lacking, yet scientific study of the particular anatomy, physiology, and function of each muscle group and their combined effort is extensive. We can make predictions based on the "average" or "normal" individual, but care must be taken in general application, because while we are all similar in our makeup, we each have our own physical variations that make us unique, and require individualization. As exercise instructors, we must present options and adaptations so our participants can proceed safely and effectively.

We start our individual exercise analysis with the hamstring group. This group is often the most important in our eyes. We seem to get the greatest amount of questions about this muscle group in our workshops.

REFERENCES

1. Fleck, S.J. and Kreamer, W. J. 1987. *Designing Resistance Training Programs*. Champaign, IL: Human Kinetics Books.

2. Westcott, W. 1989. *Strength Fitness: Physiological Principles and Training Techniques*. Dubuque, IA: Wm. C. Brown Publishers.

3. Graves, J., Welsch, M., Pollock, M. July/August 1991. Exercise Training for Muscular Strength and Endurance. *IDEA Today*, pg 33-40.

4. Lubell, A. 1989. Potentially dangerous exercises, are they harmful to all? *Phys. Sports Med*, 17:1, 187-192.

MUSCLE GROUP/JOINT STRUCTURE REVIEW

HAMSTRINGS AND GLUTEUS MAXIMUS

■ Hamstrings

Muscles

Muscle Movement & Range of Motion

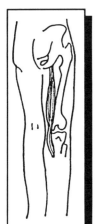 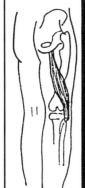 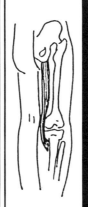 

Semi-tendinosis *Biceps femoris* *Semi-membranosis*

Origin: pelvic bone
Insertion: below the knee

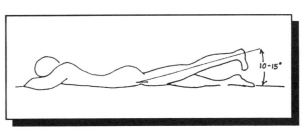

Hip hyperextension: 10-15°

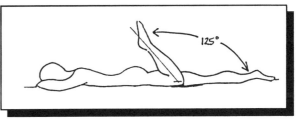

Knee flexion: 125°

■ "Gluts"

Muscles

Muscle Movement & Range of Motion

Gluteus maximus

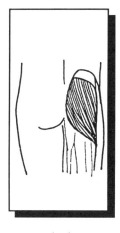

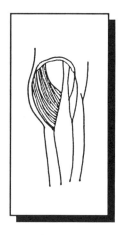

posterior view

side view

— Extends the hip (10-15°, see hamstring range of motion)
— Rotates the hip laterally (outward)

Most of the exercises that work the hamstrings group also work the Gluteus Maximus. When the hamstrings and gluts are used together, the gluts become the primary mover when hip extension exceeds 40° (of range of motion) and the knee is flexed.

■ Hamstring and Glut Stretches: CAUTION!

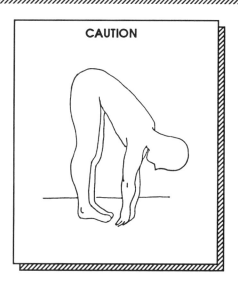

CAUTION

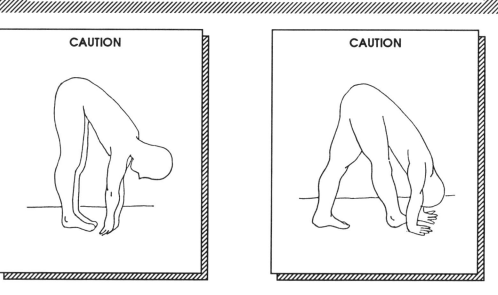

CAUTION

— This is an eccentric muscle contraction! Little flexibility gained when a muscle is contracting.
— Unsupported forward flexion past 70° stresses the low back.
— See Chapter 9 for detailed analysis.

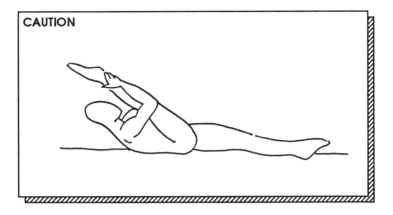

— *Beyond range of motion of hip joint (~120°). Excessive stretch of hamstrings, gluts, and hip flexors.*
— *Sciatic nerve will often give pain feedback, hamstrings will often cramp in response to excessive stretching.*
— *This much flexibility not necessary for average individuals.*

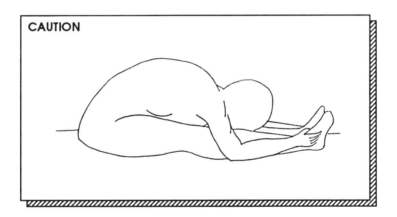

— *"All American Slouch" promotes poor posture habits.*
— *More of an upper back stretch than a hamstring stretch.*
— *See Chapter 9 for detailed analysis.*

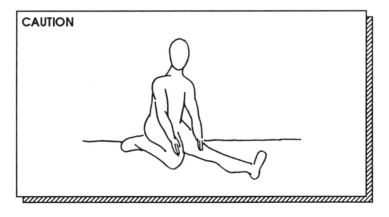

— *Unnecessary strain put on knee ligaments in turned-out knee.*

■ Hamstring and Glut Stetches: RECOMMENDED!

Progression:

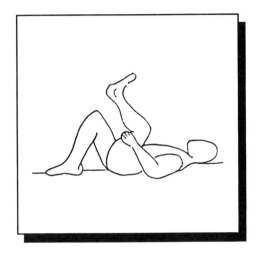

A) *Begin stretching the glut and upper hamstring.*

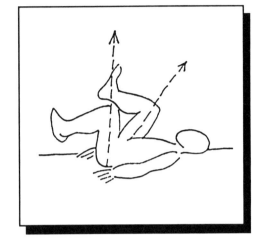

B) *Isolated glut stretch with gravity minimized.*
- *Bring one knee up at a time.*
- *Maintain 90° or greater, both legs.*

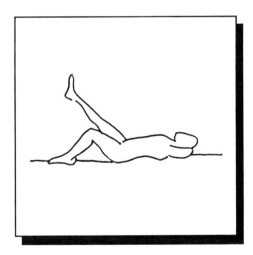

C) *Slowly start straightening out the leg. **Stop** when you feel tension or arching of back.*

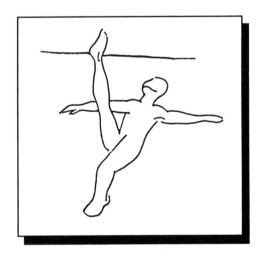

D) *Strive for a 90° lift straight up.*

— *Keep knee relaxed, never locked.*
— *Add arms below the knee on D if desired.*
— *Relax hip/back/head on the ground.*

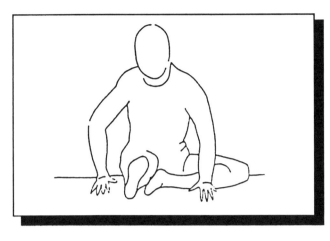

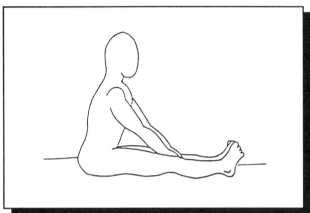

— *Use arms to support the back, to reach and return from the stretched position.*
— *Bend at the hip, and not the waist.*
— *Reach chin to toes/chest and head up.*
— *See Chapter 9 for detailed analysis.*

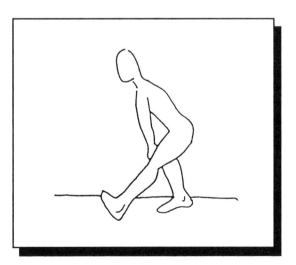

— *A good standing stretch done during warm up to prevent injury.*
— *Support the upper body with weight on the bent knee.*
— *Chin up - chest up.*
— *Tilt pelvis as if you were "mooning" the wall.*
— *Keep straight leg relaxed.*

■ Hamstring and Glut Strengthening: CAUTION!

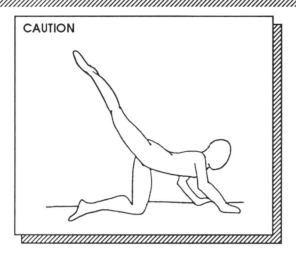

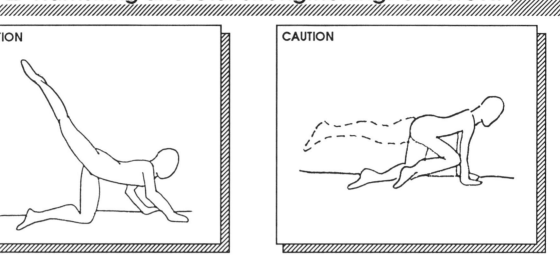

CAUTION

CAUTION

— Beyond 10-15° range of motion for hip extension.
— May compress lower lumbar discs.

— Hip flexion uses the iliospoas/quad muscle. Since these muscles are generally stronger, momentum and not deliberate muscle action will usually take over.
— Keep knees parallel, and do **not** flex knee forward to begin exercise.

■ Hamstring and Glut Strengthening: RECOMMENDED!

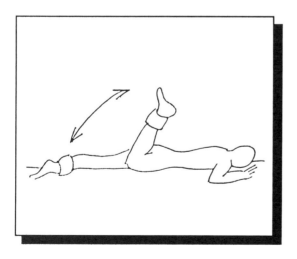

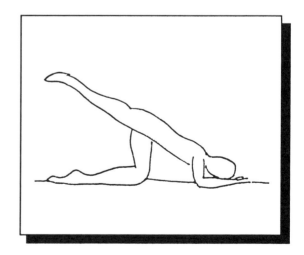

— Bend knee, moving heel towards seat for hamstring strengthening.
— May add resistance (ankle weights, rubber bands) to decrease the number of repetitions necessary for strengthening.

— Strive to maintain natural lumbar curve.
— Keep thigh and hip level.
— Compress abdominals for trunk support.
— Participants with knee pain should use the first exercise on the following page.

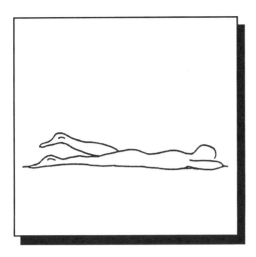

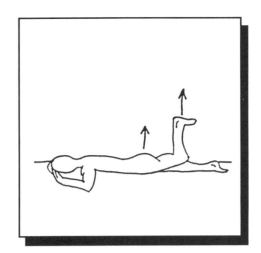

— *Keep spine in line, head relaxed on hands.*
— *Hipbones should remain on the floor.*
— *May want to use this exercise to teach proper (10-15°) range of motion.*
— *This is a strengthening exercise for the low back also.*

— *Keep the hipbones on the floor.*
— *Imagine you have strings attached to your buttocks and your foot. As the strings pull up, lift your buttocks and foot at the same time.*
— *An advanced exercise for people with back problems.*

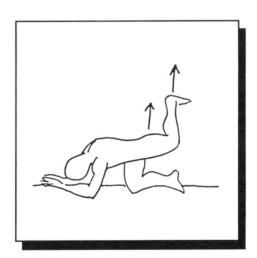

— *With the knee flexed, the gluteus maximus is the primary mover.*
— *Imagine you have a plate on your foot and you do not want to break it as you lift.*
— *Relax from the knee down; movement comes from the hip. Keep hipbones parallel to floor/pelvis stable.*

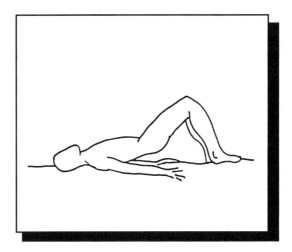

— *A largely isometric exercise, strengthens gluts, however, strengthens lower back stabilizer muscles effectively.*
— *Avoid raising hips so high that back arches, and weight is supported by head and neck - keep hips in line with knees - or lower.*
— *Is more effective for strengthening lower back muscles than working gluts, use infrequently for glut strengthening.*

CALVES

Muscles

Muscle Movement & Range of Motion

Soleus   *Gastrocnemius*

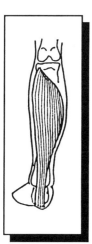   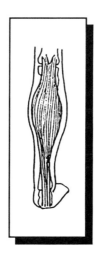

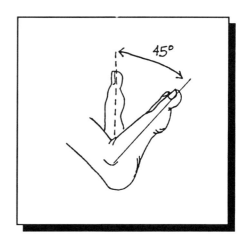

Soleus attaches below the knee.
Gastrocnemius attaches above the knee.

Plantar flexion of foot — 45°.

■ Calf Stretches: CAUTION!

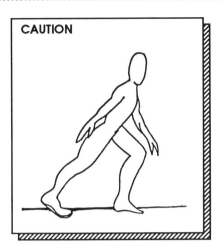

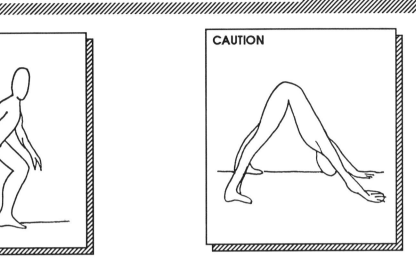

— *Back heel needs to be on the floor.*
— *Weight is shifted too far forward.*
— *If knee on front leg is bent too much (knee is past toe) the stretch may stress the ligaments of the knee.*

— *If you have inflexible hamstring muscles, this stretch may cause back pain.*
— *Using this stretch **after** the aerobic segment will cause an increase in cerebral pressure and may cause fainting because of poor blood return.*
— *Can be stressful on wrists, especially if participants have arthritis in the wrists/ hands.*

■ Calf Stretches: RECOMMENDED!

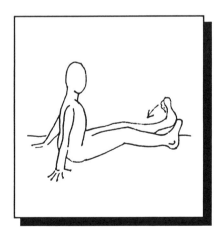

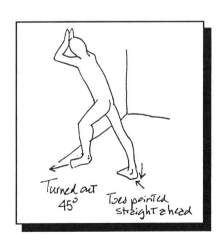

— *Straight leg on top is relaxed, and not locked.*
— *Pull toe back toward face.*
— *Support back with hands.*
— *Chest/chin are up.*
— *Reach chin to toes to maintain good posture.*

— *Back toe is pointed directly forward.*
— *Weight shifted forward.*
— *Relax back leg/heel on the floor.*
— *This stretch is effective for the gastrocnemius.*

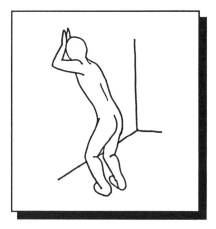

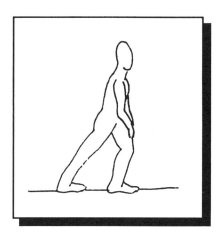

— *Heels on the floor.*
— *Both toes pointed forward/hips square.*
— *This stretch is effective for the soleus.*

— *Standing calf stretches without a wall may promote balance.*
— *Back toe should be pointed straight ahead. Front foot can be turned in or out slightly if balance is a problem.*
— *Keep torso erect - weight shifted to front leg to prevent contraction of the gastrocnemius muscle.*
— *Hands on front thigh to support torso or out to side for increased balance.*

■ Calf Strengthening

Since most walking and jogging involves the calf muscle, it is generally a strong muscle. More attention should be paid to warming up and stretching the calves than to strengthening them. Pictured below is an example of a calf strengthening/warm-up activity.

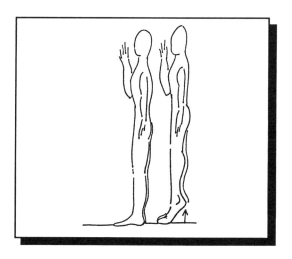

SHINS

Muscles

Anterior tibialis

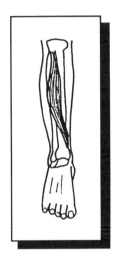

Attaches below the knee on the tibia, involves foot movement only.

Muscle Movement & Range of Motion

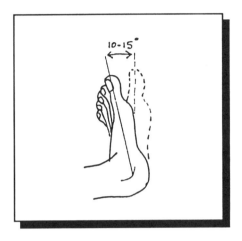

Dorsi flexion of foot — 10-15°.

> **Muscle movement note:** The anterior (front) tibialis dorsi flexes the foot, and the posterior (back) tibialis plantar flexes the foot. The posterior tibialis therefore does the same movement as the calves. Our focus on the shins will be on the anterior tibialis muscle. In terms of muscle balance, it is essential to include shin strengthening exercises in the workout, especially if the room is small or little walking is done. Brisk walking is an excellent shin strengthening exercise, however; correct walking technique should be emphasized to decrease shin stress. Initial foot strike should be on the heel, rolling foot forward and pushing off on the ball of the foot, completely extending the ankle.

■ Shin Strengthening: RECOMMENDED!

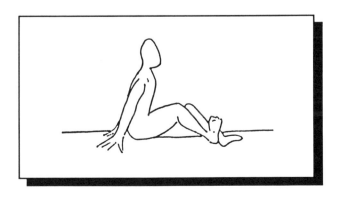

— Dorsiflex toes (1/2 time or double tempos).
— Turn toes in and out to work various range of motion.
— Ankle circles, sitting and touching toes and heels.
— Can also be accomplished standing, lying back with feet in air, or sitting in a chair.

■ Shin Stretches: RECOMMENDED!

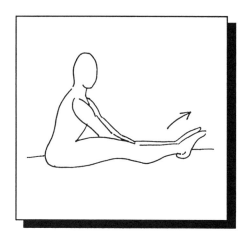

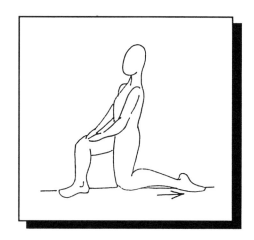

— Pointing the toes is an excellent way to stretch the shins.

— This stretch is effective for the hip flexor, quadriceps, and shin muscles.
— If participants have knee problems, perform this same stretch sitting on a chair instead.
— Keep good posture. Be sure the front knee is not flexed past the ankle.

LOWER BACK

Muscles

Spine - Erector spinae group

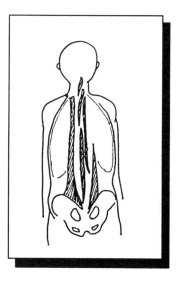

These muscles contract against gravity all day when the body is in a standing position. They should be strong muscles; however, poor posture and bending at the waist can cause these muscles to be weak.

Spinal Structure

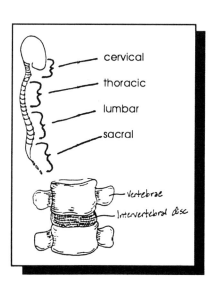

cervical
thoracic
lumbar
sacral

Vertebrae
Intervertebral disc

Between each verte-brae is a cushion or pad - the intervertebral discs. These add shock absorption and com-pressive capabilities to the spine and maintain joint spacing.

Muscle Movement & Range of Motion

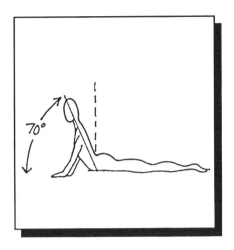 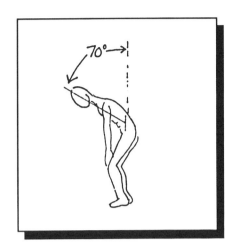

— *Hyperextends the spine 70°.*
— *Allows forward flexion of 70°.*

■ Lower Back Stretches: CAUTION!

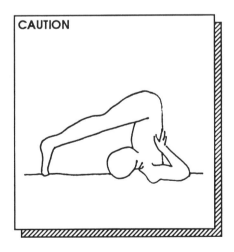

CAUTION

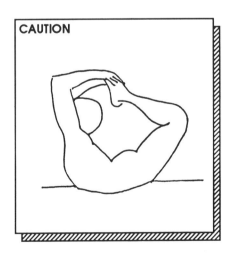

CAUTION

— *Excessive pressure on cervical spinal structures (discs, nerves and arteries).*
— *Difficult for participants with tight hamstring and back muscles.*
— *Requires strength and momentum to get into and maintain position.*
— *Hard to breathe in this position.*

— *Excessive pressure on lumbar discs.*
— *Requires hyperextension of thoracic spine (very limited) and shoulder joint.*
— *Promotes overflexibility, may be appropriate for gymnastics or other sports that require extreme spinal flexibility.*

■ Lower Back Stretches: RECOMMENDED!

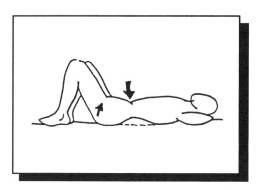

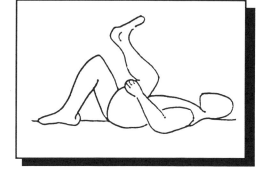

— Feet flat, knees bent, push back against floor.
— If you had a tail, tucked it between your legs and pulled, you would have the correct motion.
— Push down, hold a few seconds - keep breathing!
— Release and return to normal lumbar curve or curve that would be present with hands/towel roll in small of back.
— Important abdominal exercise as well. Abdominal muscles attached to pubis symphysis are main movers in the pelvic tilt.

— Pull one knee toward chest with hands behind the knee.
— Might aim your knee at the opposite shoulder, which will stretch with a slight twist.
— Keep head and upper back relaxed on the ground.

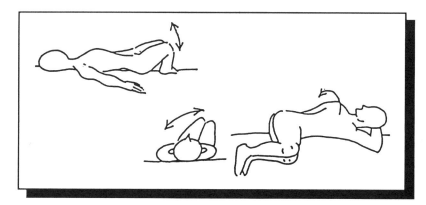

— Keep knees together.
— **Gently** drop knees to one side.
— Bring knees back to center before repeating on other side.

— Pull knees up at a 90° angle.
— Maintain curve of the spine.
— Drop one shoulder back, opening chest and face toward the ceiling.

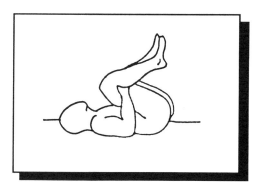

— A more advanced low back stretch.
— Pull one knee to chest, then the other. When placing feet back on floor - lower one foot, then the other.

■ Lower Back Strengthening: CAUTION!

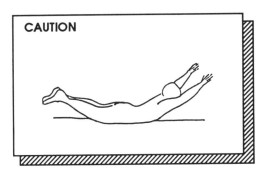

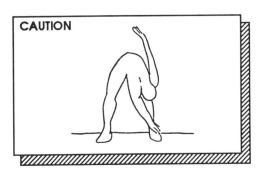

— Lifting the hands and feet at the same time increases disc pressure in the lower lumbar area.
— Often performed with speed and momentum, instead of slowly and smoothly for strengthening.
— May be used as an **advanced** back exercise for people who can perform easier exercises and maintain spinal stabilization.

— Flexion and rotation exercises put the back in the most vulnerable position for injury.
— This exercise overstretches ligaments and tendons of the back and decreases the spine's ability to withstand compressive forces.

■ Lower Back Strengthening: RECOMMENDED!

Progression:

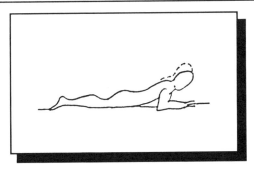

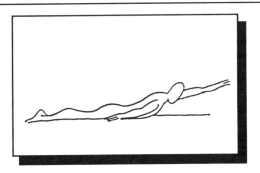

A)
— This is a **must** exercise because we need to counteract all the flexion we do in daily living.
— Push up slowly, leading with the head.
— Forearms should remain on the ground.
— Lift with back extensors, **not** by pushing up with arms and shoulders.

B)
— Lift one arm at a time or one leg at a time, slowly and with control.
— Keep the hipbones on the ground.
— Keep the upper body and head relaxed.

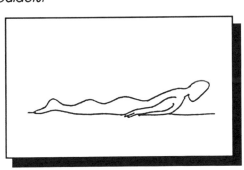

C)
— Relax the leg and glut muscles.
— **Slowly** lift the upper body up off the ground.
— This is an advanced back exercise because you are lifting the upper body without support.

ABDOMINALS

Muscles

Rectus abdominis	Transversus abdominis	Internal obliques	External obliques

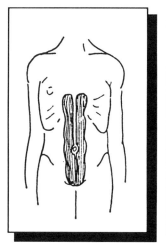 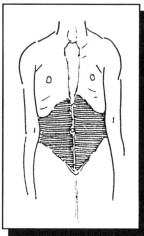 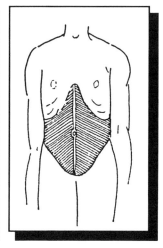 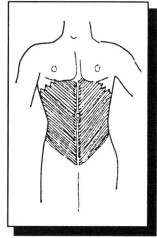

Note that there is not an "upper" or "lower" muscle. Also note the direction of striation of each of the muscles.

Muscle Movement & Range of Motion

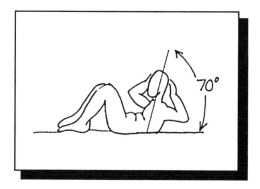

— *Flexes the spine and compresses abdominal contents. Although their full range of motion is 70°, we use smaller range of motion exercises and compression exercises for improvement of posture and spinal stabilization.*

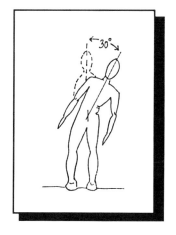

— *Laterally bends the torso to the side approximately 30°.*

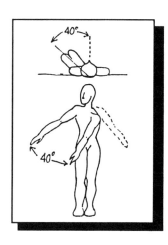

— *Rotates the torso approximately 40° with hips in a fixed position.*

■ Abdominal Stretches: RECOMMENDED!

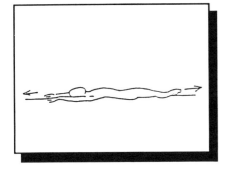

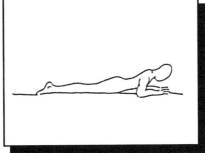

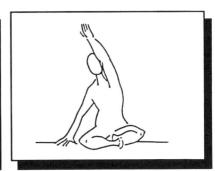

— Arch the back slightly.
— Reach with arms and point the toes.
— This is also a good stretch for the shins and hip flexor muscles.

— Lift the head up - slowly.
— Begin using back muscles only, then as you lift a little higher, support with the arms.

— Reach up with one hand and support the spine with the other hand.
— You can perform the same exercise standing, allow lower arm to slide along the leg.
— Avoid raising both arms overhead and performing lateral bends, since twisting and loss of control may result.

■ Abdominal Strengthening: CAUTION!

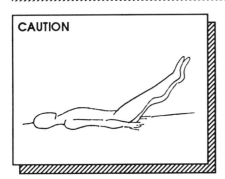
CAUTION

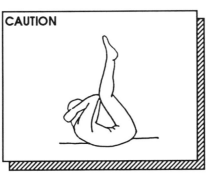
CAUTION

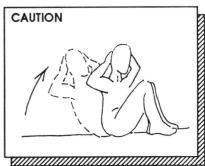
CAUTION

— Hip flexor and low back muscles perform much of the work in a double leg lift.
— Stressful on lower back, except in very strong participants who can maintain pelvic tilt and spinal stabilization.
— Detailed analysis in Chapter 9.

— Arms pulling up on the head are putting excess pressure on the cervical spine.
— Purpose of the hands behind the head is to **support** the head. Elbows out to the side is a better technique.

— Not as **effective** as alternative exercises because the hip flexors and lower back are involved.
— The phase where the individual lowers himself to the floor is the most dangerous for the low back, unless the participant carefully rolls down. Detailed analysis in Chapter 9.

■ Abdominal Strengthening: RECOMMENDED!

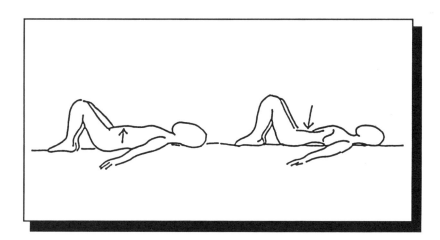

- *Abdominal compressions are important because this is how the abdominal muscles must work for sitting/ standing postures, and to stabilize and support the low back during lifting and work activities.*
- *Lie on the back with knees bent to relax the abdominal muscles.*
- *Breathe in, allowing abdominal area to rise and expand.*
- *Begin exhalation and pull abdominal muscles in as tight as possible.*
- *Continue breathing, stretching, and contracting the abdominal muscles.*
- *Slight modification could be lifting (like a curl-up) and holding for a count of four.*
- *See Chapter 4, Breathing Techniques for Standing or Sitting Compression.*

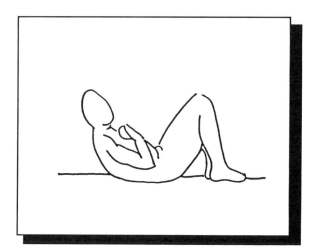

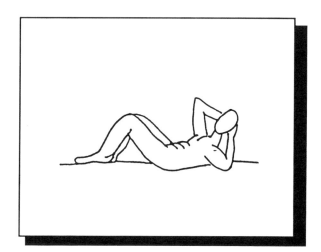

- *The further the arms are away from the abdominals, the greater the resistance.*
- *Movement should begin by curling the chin to the chest and continuing to roll until the shoulder blades have cleared the floor.*
- *Look at your knees.*
- *Use your arms to support your head if neck muscles fatigue before abdominals.*

- *This exercise works the oblique muscles predominantly.*
- *Lead with the shoulder, and not the elbow.*
- *Keep one elbow (or straight arm) on the ground to stabilize upper back muscles and ensure full range of motion.*
- *Exhale on the effort.*

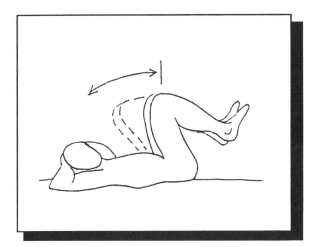

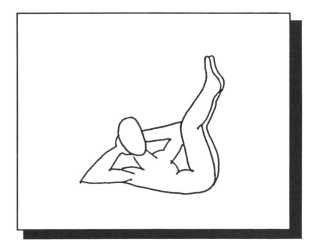

— *A reverse curl (curling the abdominals from the lower end) reverses the load. You will feel the greatest muscle contraction where the load is.*
— *Bring knees toward the chest, slowly let knees curl back.*
— *Knees must remain over the hips to keep the back flat and eliminate hip flexor involvement.*

— *Legs can be extended slightly upward.*
— *Knees are bent.*
— *Keep knees over the hips and low back.*

ABDOMINAL STRENGTHENING KEY POINTS IN REVIEW

✓ **Remember to include abdominal compression exercises in your routines. The compression exercises are the most important abdominal exercise since compression in standing, sitting, and while lifting helps stabilize the low back.**

✓ **Work the obliques by curling crosswise. The rectus abdominis gets enough work through forward flexion during daily activity. Try to include more oblique work in the abdominal segment.**

✓ **Constantly remind participants to maintain the pelvic tilt during curl-ups. Keeping the knees bent during abdominal exercises helps to maintain the pelvic tilt position. The pelvic tilt position is the key to strengthening the abdominals effectively.**

✓ **Use the pelvic tilt position and return to normal low back curve to help participants establish their position of spinal stability to be used with other exercises and activities.**

✓ **Encourage breathing. The most effective method is to exhale on the effort (while curling up).**

✓ **Watch participants' hand position behind the head. Suggest placing just fingers under the back of the head for support. Avoid jerking on the neck and keep the elbows out to the side. If you can see your elbows, they are forward, not out to the side! "Feel the weight of the head on your fingers."**

✓ **Change the "load" by doing reverse abdominal curls as well as forward flexion curl-ups.**

NECK

Muscles

Sternocleidomastoid

Levator scapulae
Iliocostalis cervicis
Longissimus capitis

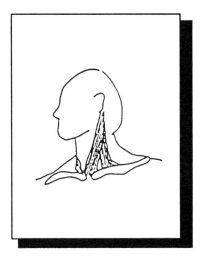

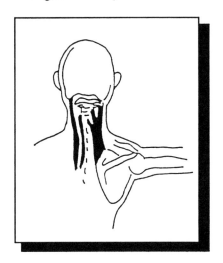

Muscle Movement & Range of Motion

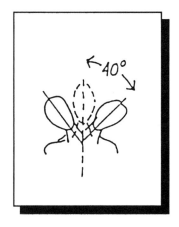

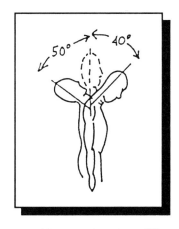

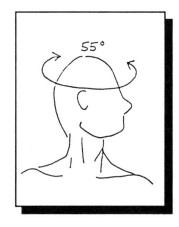

Abduction and
Adduction: 40°

Hyperextension: 50°
Flexion: 40°

Rotation: 55°

■ Neck Stretches and Strengthening: CAUTION!

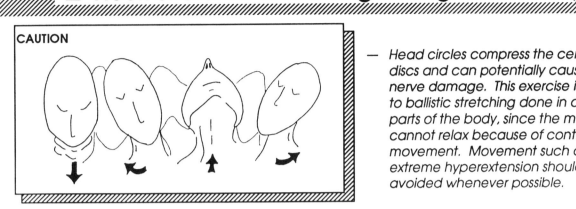

— *Head circles compress the cervical discs and can potentially cause nerve damage. This exercise is similar to ballistic stretching done in other parts of the body, since the muscles cannot relax because of continued movement. Movement such as extreme hyperextension should be avoided whenever possible.*

— *Forward neck flexion (chin to chest) is overdone in our daily activities. Emphasize other neck range of motion exercises.*

— *Hyperextension (looking up) can cause excess pressure on cervical discs and nerves, especially if performed quickly.*

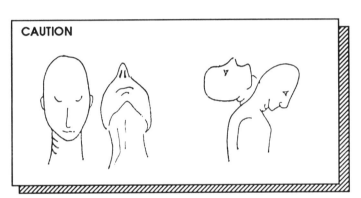

■ Neck Stretches and Strengthening: RECOMMENDED!

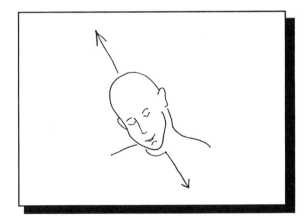

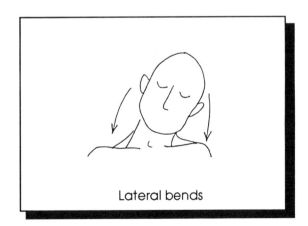

Lateral bends

— *Diagonal stretches are a comfortable change. Try using a clock face for diagonal directions. (For example, move your head so your chin is pointing at 4 o'clock, and the top of your head is at 10 o'clock.)*

— *Keep the 40° range of motion in mind when performing lateral side bends. Instructing "ear to shoulder" is anatomically impossible. Verbal directions of "side to side, shoulders down and relaxed," or "move your ear toward your shoulder," are more appropriate.*

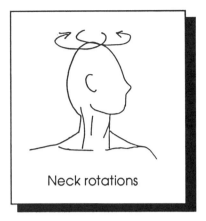

Neck rotations

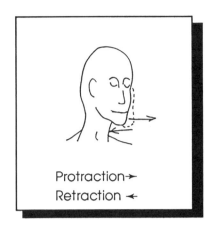

Protraction→
Retraction ←

— *"Turn your head, looking toward your shoulder." Notice the difference between the instructions - "turn your head, looking over your shoulder." Use of the word "over" may result in going past the range of motion and risk injury to the cervical spine or activation of trigger points in the neck and shoulder.*

— *Gliding the chin forward and back (like a chicken!) is an excellent exercise to counteract the effects on the neck of daily living activities.*

QUADRICEPS

Muscles

| Rectus femoris | Vastus medialis | Vastus lateralis | Vastus intermedialis |

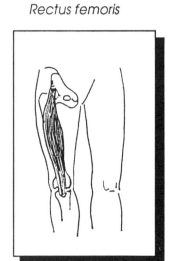
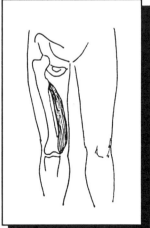
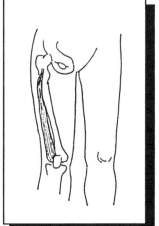
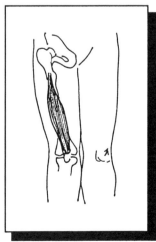

— *Rectus femoris attaches on the pelvic bone and assists the iliopsoas (not pictured) with hip flexion. The other three quad muscles (vastus medialis, vastus lateralis and vastus intermedialis) are responsible for knee extension and **not** hip flexion.*

Muscle Movement & Range of Motion

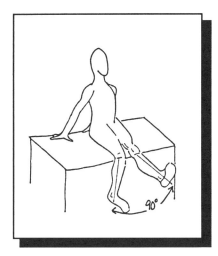

— *Knee extension: 90°*

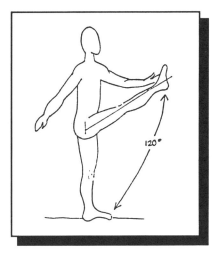

— *Hip flexion: 120°*

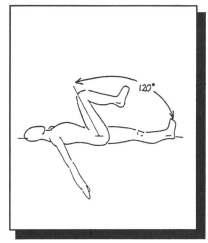

— *Hip flexion with knee flexion: 120°*

■ Quadricep Stretches: CAUTION!

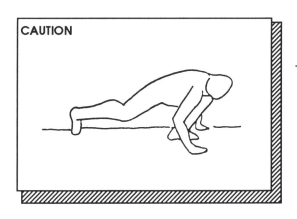

CAUTION

— *The straight leg is not relaxed against gravity, and therefore is not a passive stretch. The front knee has a great deal of strain on the ligaments.*

— *This position creates a lot of stress on the knee (patellar) ligaments, and can result in hamstring cramps or increase in back pain due to extreme positioning and precarious base of support.*

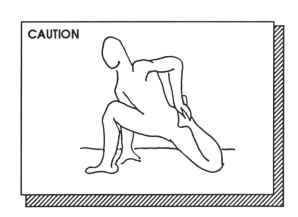

CAUTION

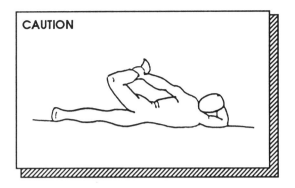

CAUTION

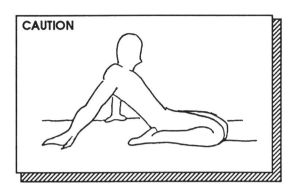

CAUTION

— Isolates the hip flexor muscle more than the quads and can cause excessive arching of the low back if not cued carefully.

— This position is extremely stressful on the knee joint. It is even more stressful on the knee joint than deep knee bends, because the upper body weight is opening up and adding pressure to the knee joint. Leaning back can also hyperextend the low back.

■ Quadricep Stretches: RECOMMENDED!

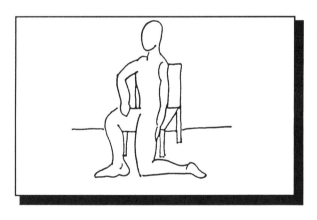

— Sit on the edge of a chair and turn to the side. Leg closest to the back of the chair goes over the side, drape arm over the back of the chair for balance. Sitting side saddle, drop free leg, knee pointing straight down at the ground. Can do this same exercise standing, without the chair, but it does add pressure to the knee joint.

— Lie relaxed, and slowly lift heel toward buttocks. This stretch will contract the hamstrings, thus relaxing the quads. Add the hand to the foot if the hamstring gets tired.

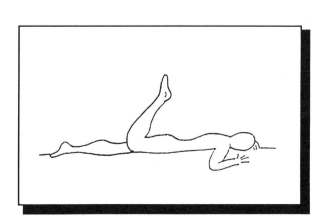

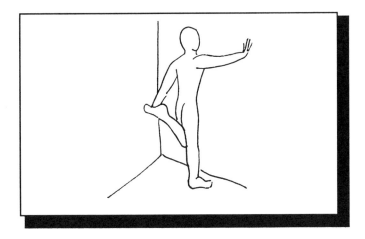

- *Relax foot in hand and* **do not** *pull to seat. Be sure knees are parallel. Maintain good posture.*
- *Use right hand and right leg, or left hand and left leg to avoid excessive twisting or rotating knee and hip outward.*

■ Quadricep Strengthening: CAUTION!

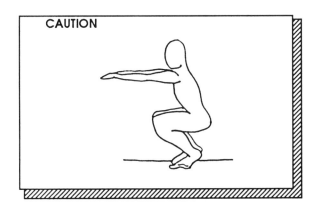

- *When you perform deep knee bends, you exert seven times your body weight on your knee joint. During exercise, never let the buttocks go below the knees.*

- *Wall sits can put too much weight and compression on the knee joint.*
- *This is an isometric exercise that will increase blood pressure and strengthen this range of motion only.* **Not** *a good exercise for downhill skiers (who skis in this position?), but sometimes used in rehab of the knee joint.*

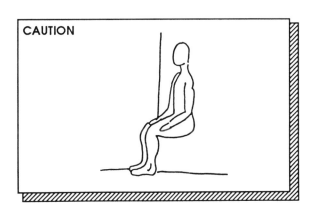

■ Quadricep Strengthening: RECOMMENDED!

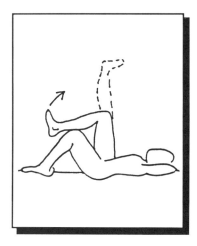 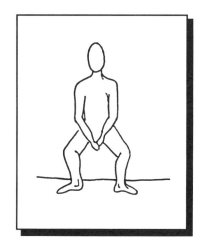 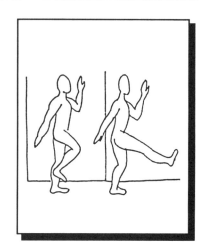

— *Slowly flex and extend the knee against gravity. There is not a lot of resistance, so this exercise is good for muscular endurance, especially with beginners.*

— *Standing in this position and bending the knees slightly uses your body weight as resistance to strengthen the quads, particularly the knee extensors.*
— *Most daily lifting takes place between knee and shoulder level. This provides good practice for daily living.*

— *Standing knee flexion is more difficult, because the hip flexor is isometrically contracting and may fatigue quicker than the quad knee extensors.*

INNER THIGH

Muscles

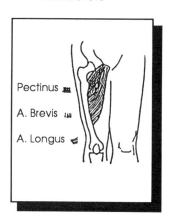

Adductors

Pectinus
A. Brevis
A. Longus

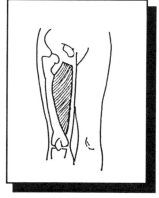

Adductor magnus

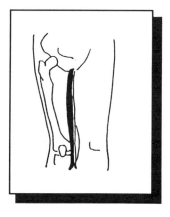

Gracilis

Adductor longus and magnus adduct and rotate the thigh laterally. Gracilis adducts, flexes, and rotates the thigh medially at the knee.

Muscle Movement & Range of Motion

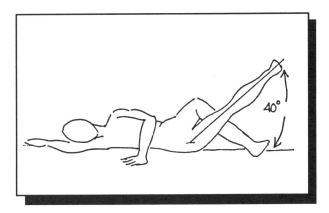

— *Adducts the thigh 40°.*
— *Assists in rotating the thigh laterally and medially.*

■ Inner Thigh Stretches: CAUTION!

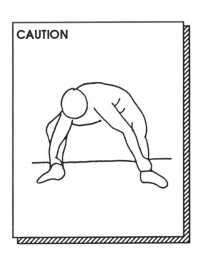

CAUTION

— *There is pressure on the hamstrings, lower back, and knees, NOT an effective stretch. The muscles are working, not passive (relaxed against gravity).*

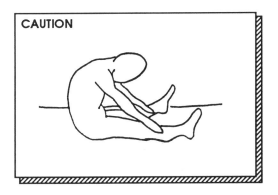

CAUTION

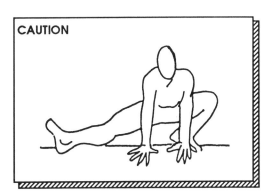

CAUTION

— *Encourages very poor posture. Discourage the "All-American Slouch" in all exercises.*

— *Overstretching of knee ligaments in the bent knee.*

■ Inner Thigh Stretches : RECOMMENDED!

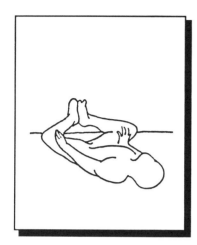

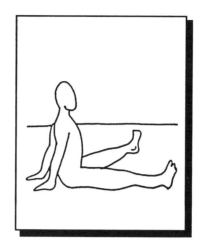

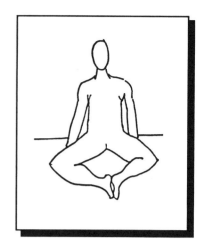

— Lie on back with seat next to a wall. Slowly slide toes down the wall until stretch is felt. If tight hip flexor muscles, press gently with hands.

— Sit up tall and push hips forward. Not necessary to bend forward from the waist. Always maintain good posture.

— Use arms to support the back. Keep head up, maintain erect spine. Relax feet and legs. Part of this exercise deals with inner thigh flexibility and part has to do with being able to externally rotate the hip. If tight hip flexors or external rotation are a problem, use the first two stretches.

■ Inner Thigh Strengthening: CAUTION!

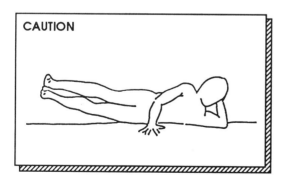

CAUTION

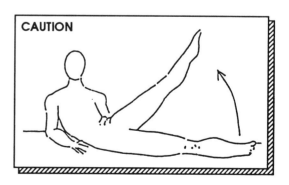

CAUTION

— The body does not have an appropriate base of support in this exercise. Because of the long lever created by the straightened legs, there will be increased intervertebral disc pressure of the back. The person might also end up **lifting** in a twisted position, increasing the risk of injury.

— The quads will end up performing much of the work in this exercise, because once the bottom leg is past 40°, the quads will continue the movement.
— The base of support is the hip, which can be very unstable. Propping the upper body on the arm is hard on the shoulder, neck, and back.

■ Inner Thigh Strengthening : RECOMMENDED!

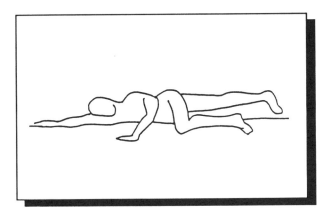

— Relax head on arm, and lift straight leg **leading with heel.**
— Note that stress to the lower back from the weight of the top leg can be painful in some individuals. Always give an option.

— Putting the top leg behind does open up the hips, but allows for a greater range of motion during strengthening, particularly for participants with larger thighs. The back may be slightly twisted, however there is less pressure from gravity on the back when lying down.
— Top leg in front will help stretch the hip and buttocks, which may help some people with back and hip problems.

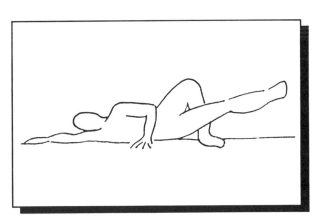

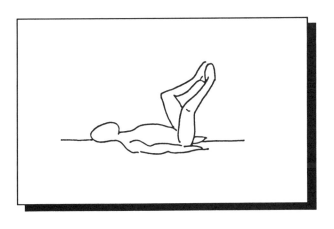

— Soles or sides of feet together, with knee over hips and back pressed flat. Glide legs up and down, emphasizing adducting the thigh. Alternative exercises would be preferred if participants have inflexible hip flexors, lower back, or hamstring muscles.

OUTER THIGH

Muscles

Gluteus medius
Tensor fasciae latae
Iliotibial tract

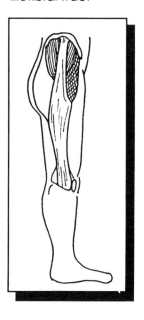

Muscles located on hip predominantly.
Iliotibial tract is composed of fascia
(connective tissue).

Muscle Movement & Range of Motion

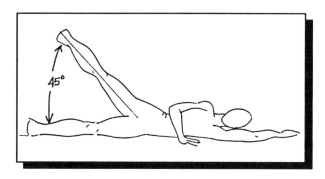

— Gluteus medius: abducts thigh 45°,
  and keeps the hips stable when you
  walk or run.
— Tensor fasciae latae: adducts,
  flexes and rotates thigh medially.

■ Outer Thigh Stretching: RECOMMENDED!

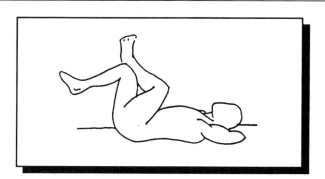

— Relax spine on the ground and place opposite ankle on the knee.
— Bring one knee over torso at a time to avoid pull on the low back.
— Keep supporting knee at 90° or less (over torso).

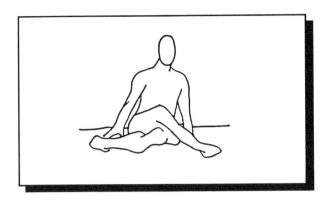

— Cross one leg in front. Maintain erect posture and relax. Support spine with hands.

■ Outer Thigh Strengthening: CAUTION!

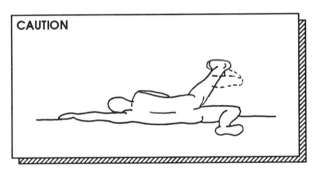

CAUTION

— The "L-position" (particularly with the leg straight) isolates the outer thigh muscles - which will fatigue quickly.
— If used at all, use a limited number of repetitions (8 or less) to minimize muscle ischemia, stress on the hip capsule, and pull on the low back.

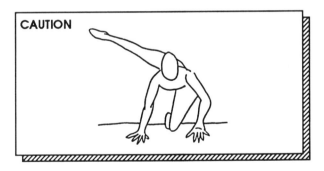

CAUTION

— Lifting the leg too high in the "doggie" position rotates the hips, and can put stress on the lower back and supporting hip, especially if the leg is straight.
— Having knees close together accentuates the twisting and leaning movement even more.
— This position can also be detrimental to participants with knee or wrist problems.

CAUTION

— If you lift beyond the 45° range of motion, the quads will be utilized. The quads are generally strong, so encourage proper range of motion (45°). Higher is **not** better!

■ Outer Thigh Strengthening: RECOMMENDED!

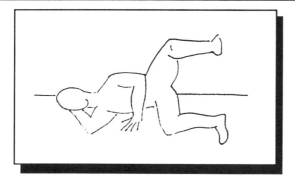

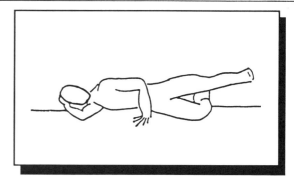

— Begin exercises with knee bent (shorter lever=less work) and progress to straightening the leg. Always allow beginners to continue with the knee bent.
— Bend the bottom leg and support with hand in front.
— Rest head on arm to keep spine relaxed, heel leads the lift. Try not to lift with "toe up," because this technique works the quadriceps.
— See Chapter 9 for detailed analysis.

— Lie on the side with bottom leg bent and top arm on ground for a good base of support.
— Relax head on bottom arm.
— Relax lifting leg from the knee down with toe facing forward or slightly down. Lift to 45°.

■ INNER AND OUTER THIGH KEY POINTS IN REVIEW

✓ Use the side lying position to work the outer thigh rather than the hands and knees position, unless your participants are advanced. The hands and knees position is harder to perform properly.

✓ In the side lying position keep the top arm in front, and when lying on the side, bend the bottom leg to keep the body from rolling forward or back. Rolling forward or back increases the likelihood of working the quads and stressing the lower back.

✓ Proper instruction for hands and knees position is "hands under shoulders and knees under hips form a better base of support. Lift no more than 45°." In the hands and knees position, alternate sides often because the supporting leg is contracting isometrically to hold the body in position.

✓ A body alignment check should be incorporated into your specific exercise. Side lying position - keep spine in line. In hands and knees position if person lifts right arm and left leg he/she remains balanced.

✓ Lifting with a straight leg increases the lever and weight, thereby increasing the work. Many participants then recruit other muscle groups to accomplish the task. Bend the knee to shorten the lever with beginners.

✓ The outer thigh (gluteus medius) is a small muscle. Do not spend a great deal of time doing outer thigh work. Performing many of these exercises continue to promote the idea of "spot reducing."

DELTOIDS

Muscles

Deltoid
(anterior view)

Deltoid
(posterior view)

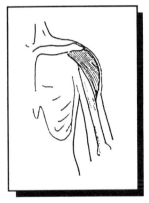 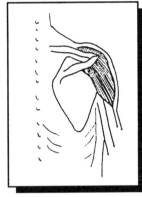

— There are three different areas of the deltoid muscle: the anterior, middle, and posterior sections. Each section has its own muscle action.

Muscle Movement & Range of Motion

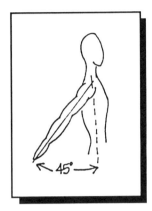 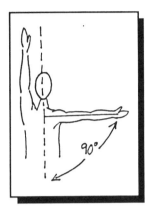

— Posterior: extends, hyperextends, and laterally rotates the shoulder joint. Hyperextension range of motion is 45°.

— Middle: abducts the shoulder joint, especially from 90-180°.
— Anterior: flexes and medially rotates the shoulder joint.

■ Deltoid Stretching: RECOMMENDED!

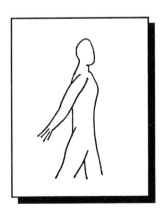

— Pull shoulders back and maintain good posture. Clasping hands is optional. Always gradually increase the range of motion of shoulder joint exercises in the warm up.

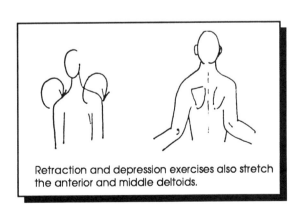

Retraction and depression exercises also stretch the anterior and middle deltoids.

— Reverse shoulder rolls performed in a slow and controlled manner are a good warm up for rotator cuff muscles, as well as a nice stretch for chest muscles and levator scapula muscles used in daily activities.

■ Deltoid Strengthening: RECOMMENDED!

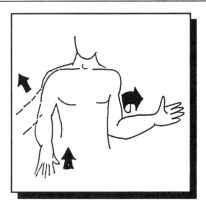

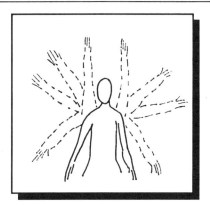

— Using all forms of the muscle's movement (flexion, extension, abduction, and hyperextension) is the most effective way to strengthen all sections of the deltoid muscle.

— Concentrate on using full range of motion movements. Remember: smaller movements strengthen through a limited range of motion and cause muscle ischemia. Try to use different planes and a fuller range of motion.

LATISSIMUS DORSI

Muscles

Muscle Movement & Range of Motion

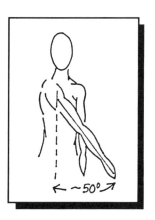

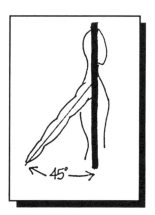

— Tend to be weak muscles because gravity pulls arms down.

Hyperabduction of the shoulder joint, range of motion is 50°.

— Assists deltoid in hyperextension of the shoulder joint, range of motion is 45°.

— Assists in lateral trunk flexion and depresses shoulder girdle.

■ Latissimus Dorsi Stretching: RECOMMENDED!

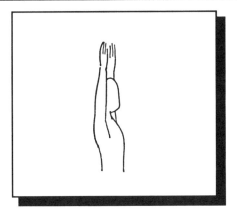

— *The "pencil stretch" whether performed lying down, standing, or sitting is an effective "lat" stretch.*

— *Reach one arm up at a time.*
— *Support upper body weight with one hand on the ground.*

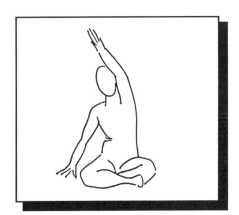

■ Latissimus Dorsi Strengthening: RECOMMENDED!

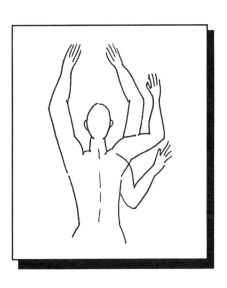

— *Reach both arms up, slowly pull arms down and slightly back. Be sure to perform this exercise in a slow and controlled manner, especially if using hand weights.*

UPPER BACK—RHOMBOIDS AND TRAPEZIUS

Muscles

Muscle Movement & Range of Motion

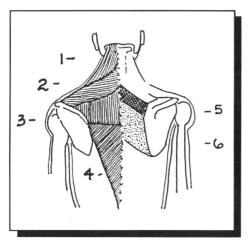

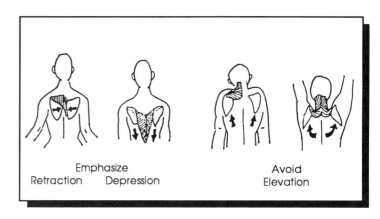

— 1-4 Trapezius
— 5 Rhomboid minor
— 6 Rhomboid major
Upper trapezius tend to be stretched muscles, due to the "All-Amercian Slouch." Lower trapezius muscles get very tight and often are areas of trigger points or muscle spasms for many people.

— We need to emphasize depression and retraction exercises to counteract shoulder elevation caused by stress, badly designed work areas, and poorly adjusted seating.

■ **Upper Back—Rhomboids and Trapezius Stretching: RECOMMENDED!**

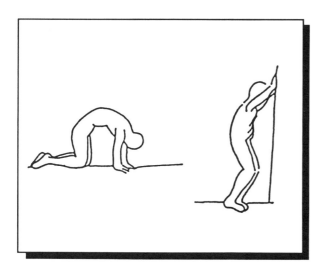

— The "cat stretch" performed standing or on hands and knees is very effective.
— Begin by taking a deep breath. As you exhale, compress the abdominals and continue the movement by arching and lifting the back and dropping the head. When a breath is needed - inhale and relax by lowering back and raising the head.
— This position is a very effective way of teaching proper breathing techniques.
— For those with knee and wrist problems, the cat stretch can be done in a standing position.

■ Upper Back—Rhomboids and Trapezius Strengthening: RECOMMENDED!

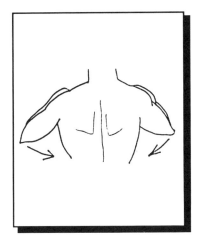 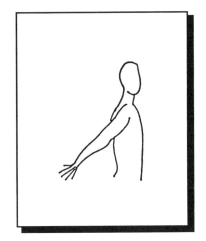 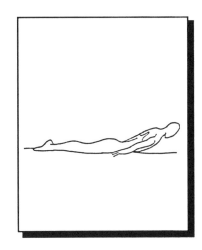

— With bent arms, press the elbows straight back, squeezing the shoulder blades together.

— With arms straight, pull back and squeeze the shoulder blades together.

— Lying flat, relax the buttocks - lift and squeeze shoulder blades together.
— This exercise also strengthens the lower back. It can be hard on the hipbones and groin areas, be sure you have appropriate padding.

CHEST—PECTORALS

Muscles

Muscle Movement & Range of Motion

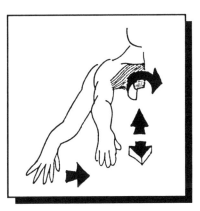

— Pectoralis major

— Adducts arm and extends shoulder.
— Acts with the anterior deltoid in horizontal flexion and medial rotation of the upper arm.

■ Chest—Pectoral Stretches: RECOMMENDED!

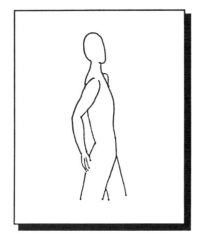 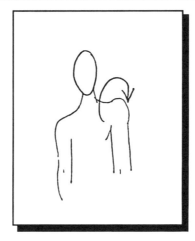 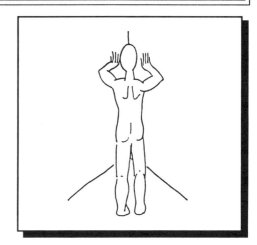

— *Press the arms back and chest forward. Maintain good posture.*

— *Reverse shoulder rolls are a good warm up/stretch for the pectorals.*

— *The corner push-up is a maximal stretch for the pectorals.*
— *Place hands on either side of the corner - hold body taut and lean into the corner until you feel a comfortable stretch, and hold.*
— *This is difficult to do in a group, since corner locations are limited, but is good to have as part of an exercise circuit.*

■ Chest—Pectoral Strengthening: RECOMMENDED!

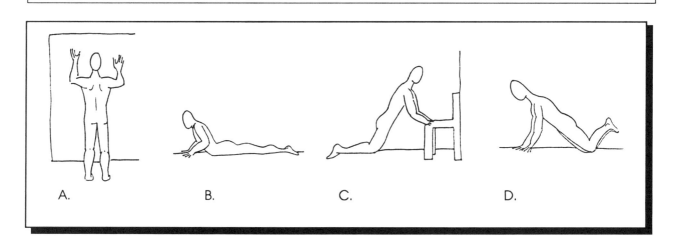

A.   B.   C.   D.

Do not expect participants to be able to lift their whole body weight immediately. Progress from (A) wall push-ups., (B) press-ups, (C) chair or step push-ups, and (D) bent knee push-ups. Unless you are teaching an advanced class or have a participant that needs a challenge and can accomplish the other types of push-ups, we do not recommend performing full or "men's" push-ups.

BICEPS AND TRICEPS

Muscles

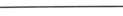

Biceps

Triceps

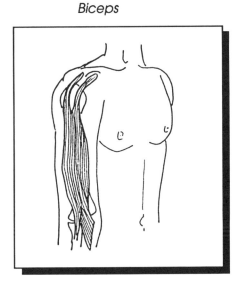
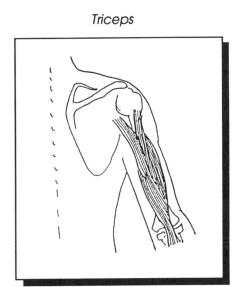

Muscle Movement & Range of Motion

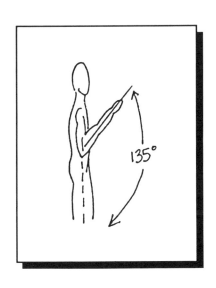

— Biceps: Flex the elbow and assist in shoulder joint flexion.
— Triceps: Extend the elbow and assist in shoulder joint extension.

135°

■ Biceps/Triceps Stretches: RECOMMENDED!

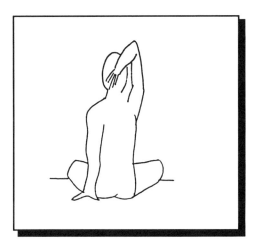

To stretch the bicep: Simply straighten out the arm. The picture above shows a tricep stretch. Be aware that putting pressure on the elbow joint can cause overstretching of the rotator cuff muscles.

■ Biceps/Triceps Strengthening: RECOMMENDED!

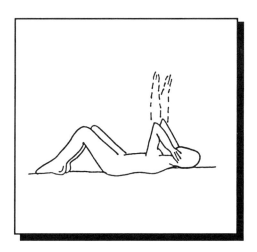

— *We do not have a picture of bicep strengthening, because the biceps are utilized in our daily activities. It is more important to strengthen the triceps.*
— *Use gravity as resistance . Keep the elbows stationary (pointed straight up at the ceiling), and close together to relax the shoulder joint.*

MUSCULAR STRENGTH/ENDURANCE/STRETCHING—PART 2

Now that we have completed the analysis of each individual muscle group, we will generally evaluate the entire muscular strength/flexibility segment. These sections are included in the overall Instructor Evaluation Tool.

VERBAL CUES ON POSTURE/ALIGNMENT

■ Since eight out of every ten Americans will have back problems during their lifetime, it is essential that you teach your entire class posture and alignment in every movement and position.

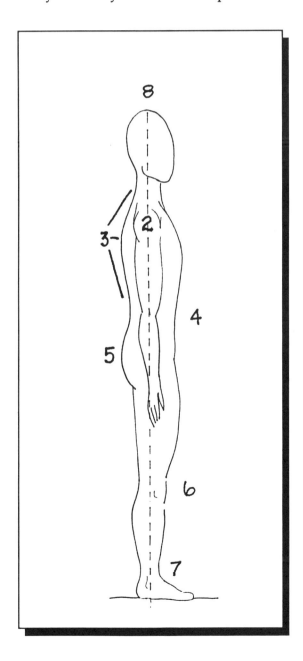

■ In a standing position:

1. Head should be suspended — not pushed back or dropped forward.
2. Arms should be suspended and hanging from the shoulder. Have people circle shoulders back and down—arms should hang at lowest point.
3. Maintain the three curves of the spine. Loss of the low back curve decreases the amount of compression the spine can withstand.
4. Lightly compress the abdominal muscles to help support the spinal column, especially with lifting. Compression helps to distribute weight over the entire torso, not just the low back. Extreme compression, however, restricts breathing.
5. Hips can be tucked slightly, particularly for sway back individuals, pregnant women, and people with a large protruding abdominal area.
6. Knees should be unlocked or soft. Locked knees shift the pelvis, contributing to an increased low back curve and back strain; along with decreased blood flow to and from the legs.
7. Feet should be shoulder width apart, weight evenly distributed. People who roll their feet to the inner or outer edges need to concentrate on keeping their weight over the entire bottom surface of each foot.
8. An imaginary plumb line dropped from the head should pass through the cervical and lumbar vertebrae, the hips, knees, and ankles.

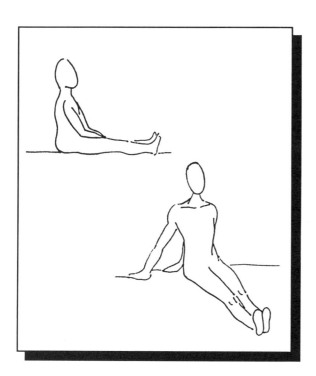

■ *In a sitting position:*

When sitting in any position, the three back curves need to be maintained.

If people cannot sit without slouching forward or backward, they need to support themselves with their hands and arms or lean against a wall or chair back.

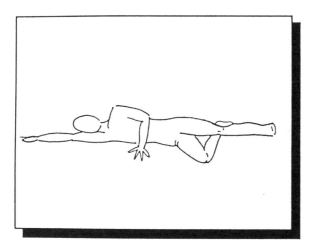

■ *In a lying position:*

In a side lying position — the spine still needs to be kept in line. Avoid propping head or upper body up on an arm and hand. Propping compromises the neck, shoulders, arms, wrists, and hands. Head should remain relaxed. Legs should be together, the leg closest to floor should have a knee bent to prevent rolling forward or backward.

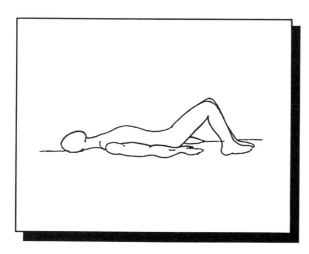

■ *In a supine position:*

Head should remain relaxed. Many people imitate their instructor by holding their heads up. Remind people that this is not necessarily a part of the exercise.

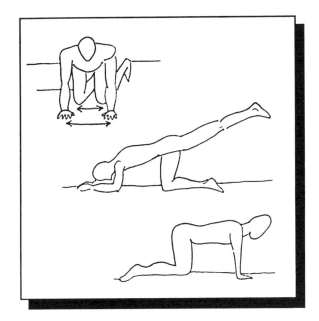

■ *Hands and knees position:*

Knees should be positioned directly under the hips, hands directly under the shoulder joints. Knees have a way of drifting close together as an exercise progresses. Remind people often that their knees should be hip width apart, and hands are shoulder width apart. People should be able to balance without falling to one side or the other. Maintain back curves — do not force the low back curve into an extreme position by pushing down . . . or by dropping on belly and raising head. . . In some exercises, participants can drop down to their forearms to keep spine in line or relieve pressure on hands/wrists.

ENCOURAGES AND DEMONSTRATES PROPER BODY MECHANICS

■   It is the obligation of the exercise instructor to *always* encourage and instruct participants in the methods of good body mechanics. First, the exercise instructor must *always* demonstrate and use good body mechanics him/herself. Most often participants will imitate you and model themselves after your example, so you have to be correct. You have many opportunities to demonstrate correct lifting (picking up a mat or exercise equipment), and using weight shifts and legs instead of the back during transitional position changes (getting up and down from the floor).

The rules of safety are simple enough, but not necessarily easy to accomplish.

RULE 1.

Keep the back as STRAIGHT as possible.

RULE 2.

MAINTAIN the CURVES of the spine, particularly in a sitting or standing position.

RULE 3.

AVOID BENDING at the waist in a standing or sitting position, bend at the hips instead. Use hands and arms for support. Without using HAND/ARM SUPPORT you end up being suspended by the back structures, and lifting with the back muscles, which is inappropriate.

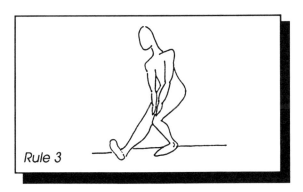

Rule 3

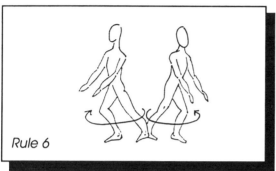

Rule 6

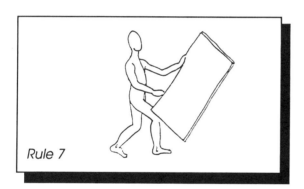

Rule 7

RULE 4.

AVOID TWISTING past the spine's range of motion in a loaded position (sitting, standing, or with added weight).

RULE 5.

Never bend at the waist and twist at the same time. Bending at the waist decreases the spine's compressive capability. Twisting has the potential to injure or tear the vertebral discs.

RULE 6.

PIVOT your whole body instead of twisting!

RULE 7.

ALWAYS, ALWAYS LIFT WITH THE LEGS! To try to lift with the back by bending over at the waist and keeping legs straight — even for a light item — is idiotic at best! The lifting capacity of back muscles is approximately 600 pounds per square inch. The lifting capacity of the legs is approximately 4000 pounds per square inch. By the way — using 4000 lbs. is not overkill! Holding a two-pound weight about two feet from the body exerts approximately 200 pounds of compressive force on the low back. Don't forget about the forces of gravity, and the weight of body parts. (Your head weighs about 12 pounds!)

RULE 8.

Create a good base of support for lifting and weight shifts by placing feet in a front to back stance. Head up. Maintain back curves.

RULE 9.

Be as careful putting objects down as when you are lifting. The further the object is from the body, greater strength and control are required. Use abdominal compression for spinal support.

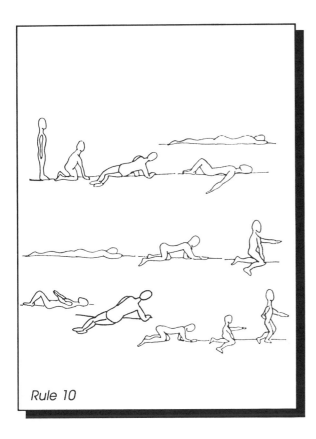

Rule 10

You need to give these instructions in each and every class. These instructions remind people over and over again about the importance of posture, positioning and body mechanics. Instructing others also keeps your own posture and body mechanics correct!

INSTRUCTS/ENCOURAGES BREATHING TECHNIQUE

■　Since we have previously discussed breathing technique in other sections of this book, we will not go into detail here. However, please remember that during floor exercise many people hold their breath while they try to crank out 10 more repetitions. Instead of making a particular movement easier, holding the breath makes an exercise more difficult by decreasing blood flow to the working muscle, and thereby increasing blood pressure. Many calisthenic or

floor exercises already have an isometric component when the exercise is initiated, which increases pressure within the cardiovascular system. Breath holding or inhaling compounds the pressure problem as well as adding to the workload, because it increases the number of muscles needed to accomplish the task. Have people take a breath before initiating a movement, and exhale as that movement progresses through the range of motion.

OBSERVES PARTICIPANTS' FORM AND SUGGESTS ADAPTATIONS FOR INJURIES/SPECIAL NEEDS

■　One of the most important differences between the "performance" instructor and the performance educator is that the educator can and will help people with their individual needs to make exercise safer and less painful or problematic. In order to facilitate this, the instructor must know the problems/limitations of his/her participants and *observe* what the participants are doing. The following story is a classic example of what can happen if you do not circulate and observe your participants as they perform their activities.

Deb worked with a client after his back surgery. He was instructed in the same body mechanics and back safety techniques that we have presented earlier in this chapter. After his recovery he returned to his regular exercise class, but continued to have back pain and difficulty, even though he felt he had analyzed the situation. Deb went to his exercise class, just to observe what might be happening (as a side note — she did inform the instructor of her presence, purpose for being there, and asked permission to observe). Everything went well during the class, however there were two or three exercises that Deb was able to identify that were the cause of his continuing difficulty.

The exercise instructor was an extremely competent educator. Her demonstration and cuing of each exercise was excellent. She also looked around during each exercise to see whether anyone was having difficulty, but she did have a large class that filled an entire gymnasium, so it is reasonable to assume that she could not observe everyone simultaneously. Even in a visual sweep of the class, she might have been observing at the wrong angle.

The two offending exercises were ones commonly used in most classes — the sit and reach hamstring stretch, and curl-ups with the knees pulled up to the chest, feet off of the floor. Deb's client, even though educated, did not have the body sense to be able to tell his deviations from his instructor's, therefore he continued to pull and irritate back muscles every time he performed these two exercises. Below are pictures of the demonstrated exercise, the deviations, and suggestions for modification.

The point of this example is not to scare you, but to *get you out on the floor—observing and assisting!* Perform a few repetitions, then get up and begin watching your participants' technique. You'll never know what is happening unless you look! In a particularly large class you may still miss a few things, so we suggest that you have some assistance — another instructor, or a student trained in exercise who can troubleshoot, or lead while you troubleshoot. An interesting result of the visit to the exercise class was that as Deb conferred with her client and the exercise instructor (at her request), three to four other class participants joined this impromptu conference, said they were having similar problems, and were happy to learn the modifications.

Sit and reach hamstring stretch:

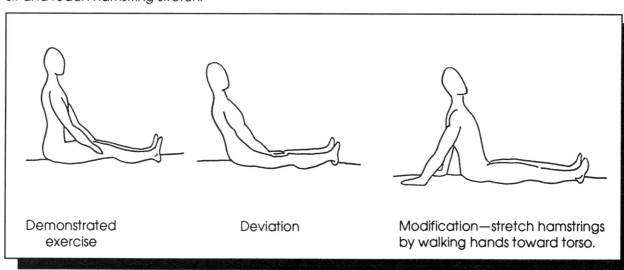

Demonstrated
exercise

Deviation

Modification—stretch hamstrings
by walking hands toward torso.

Curl-ups—Variation: knees to chest, feet off of floor

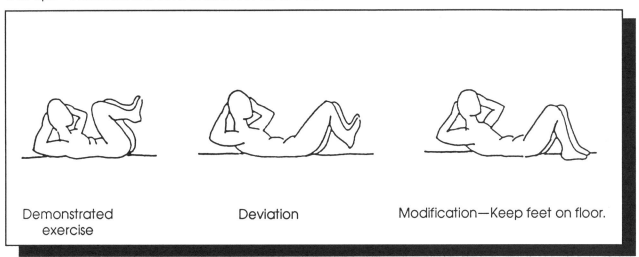

Demonstrated exercise

Deviation

Modification—Keep feet on floor.

Let's look at some other examples of modification:

Sometimes the suggestions will be quick and simple: "If placing your wrist in the hyperextended position bothers you (a), make a fist to keep your wrist rigid (b), or get down on your forearms (c)."

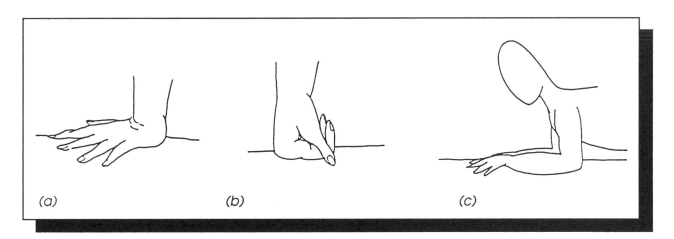

(a)

(b)

(c)

Sometimes the modifications may require less weight bearing : "If knee push-ups are too difficult (a or b) — stand up and do wall push-ups instead (c)."

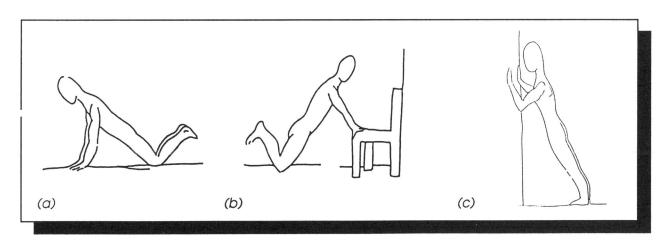

(a)

(b)

(c)

Or a change in level: "If being on your hands and knees is painful (a), try this exercise in a standing position instead (b)." Periodically you may have to confer with someone who has more training or experience with a particular problem before you can come up with the right alternative.   In this case, you might have to instruct the participant to "sit this one out" or "perform another exercise in its place" until you get the information and assistance you need.

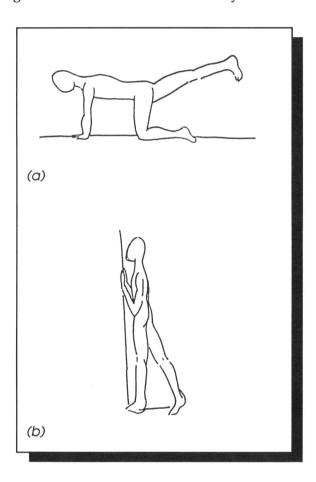

(a)

(b)

CORRECTS/RECOMMENDS CHANGES IN POLITE, NON-THREATENING WAY

■   Once you have observed a problem, you must take action. Most instructors do not feel comfortable correcting technique, but there are ways that you can correct someone's technique without being threatening or critical. Below are some suggestions for arranging and cuing the participant on correct position or technique.

General statements to the whole exercise group

"Stop for just a moment — look at your back foot to see if your toe is facing straight ahead. The toe must be straight ahead to stretch effectively." Or, "I see people having difficulty - let me demonstrate what I want you to do…"

Make corrections by moving the person into the proper position

During a wall stretch for the calves approach people having difficulty following instruction: "I am going to turn your foot so it is straight. Can you feel a difference in the stretch now?"

Exercise next to your participant

Stand beside the person having trouble and demonstrate what you want him/her to do. Perhaps they cannot quite see or hear you well enough to comply. If the person you are correcting is down on the floor - *get down* next to him/her to demonstrate. A person on the floor is more vulnerable than the person standing, therefore you must get down on the same level to instruct in a non-threatening way.

Take someone off to the side for a quick demonstration

If you do so, make sure the rest of the class is occupied, so their attention is not focused on this individual. If the only available space is a corner, position yourself there and let the participant stand closer to the room. If someone feels "cornered" and vulnerable, they will not pay much attention to what you have to offer.

Catch people doing "it" right

Most people respond much better to positive rather than negative reinforcement. If they are having difficulty with a movement or series of movements, point out someone performing well in class for them to watch or pair them together. Always demonstrate and instruct correct technique — people know how to do things the wrong way, and they often concentrate on what is wrong, *not* what is correct.

Always appeal to a person's need for safety and give your rationale

Compare the following statements:

"You must have your foot in this position."

"Place your foot in this position. It will prevent you from falling forward, and will make this exercise easier."

"Don't bounce while stretching, that's the wrong technique."

"If you bounce while stretching you might pull or tear a muscle—I don't want you to get hurt. Try holding the stretch instead."

Which would you rather hear? The second and fourth statements do not differ remarkably; however, they include a rationale and helpful alternatives.

Use positive descriptions, rather than labels

Words such as "good," "bad," "right," and "wrong" are emotionally loaded and judgmental. Instead of saying: "Joe, you are doing this movement wrong." Try "Joe, you seem to be having trouble with this movement, let's try this...I think it will help."

When all else fails, get down on your knees, then beg

We are not opposed to humor, teasing, or begging. You can obtain a lot of performance and excellence by wheedling, cajoling and begging. *You do have to know your participants though*, in order to perceive who can take ribbing and who cannot. A large part of your class is very delicately "exercising" their self-image, and increasing risk taking. Be careful. Be considerate when you are having fun — and if you feel you have offended someone, apologize.

EQUIPMENT IS USED SAFELY AND EFFECTIVELY

■ In this section we will cover information for *portable* resistance training equipment that you might use in your class — rubber bands, surgical tubing, balls, hand and ankle weights, ropes, dowels, frisbees, hula-hoops, and other "stuff" that you may use to make your classes varied and fun. We will not be addressing use of any free weights (other than dumbbells), weight machines, or par courses, since the techniques used for weight training are beyond the scope of this book.

If you will be using weightlifting equipment in your class, we recommend that you become very knowledgeable about the type of machinery you will be using. You should actually try each machine and exercise(s), learn the adjustments for people of different dimensions, ways the machinery can be adapted, if at all, and look at the body mechanics that must be used to get in and out of the machine, as well as during its use. We would like to suggest that you apply the principles of the SEARCH tool, as well as the information previously covered in this chapter to analyze the safety and effectiveness of each machine.

While all manufacturers and distributors would have you believe their machines or weights are "the best," and cover all of your participants' needs, YOU need to evaluate those claims and the risk to benefit for your participants. For example, several manufacturers of weightlifting devices have machines for abduction/adduction of the legs and back extension. In analyzing weightlifting devices, remember the muscles and other structures that work the inner and outer thigh. Analyze the need to strengthen these areas versus the public desire to spot reduce. Is the machine really helpful or does it continue to mislead and misinform the participants about what their bodies actually need and can do?

Even within the pages of this book we have suggested use of hyperextension exercises for strengthening the back; but consider that we suggest exercises that minimize gravity, and allow the spine to be "unloaded" or non-weightbearing. Most machines have the person working on hyperextension, with the spine in a loaded or weightbearing position. There is nothing wrong with that necessarily— except that this would be an advanced part of any back strengthening progression, not a beginning exercise.

We discourage the use of hand-held weights or resistance devices during the aerobic segment. Several research studies document the fact that the addition of one or two pounds of weight *does not* significantly increase the energy expended at that time (1,2). Furthermore, it has been our experience that use of hand or ankle weights greatly increases the risk of injury by decreasing control or changing movement patterns significantly. We prefer to make a distinct separation between the strengthening and cardiopulmonary segment of a class. It is appropriate to use weights and resistive devices during the muscular strengthening and endurance portion of the class.

Let's look at some of the "portable" strength training equipment that you may use in your general exercise or floor work-out class, and some safety guidelines that we have found to be important.

■ PORTABLE STRENGTHENING EQUIPMENT

Rubber band:	These are bigger versions of your typical rubber bands. They come in different thicknesses or sizes so that there can be a progression of work. The thicker the band, the greater the work. Placed around two body parts, or a body part and an object (the legs of a chair), the bands provide resistance for increased strengthening. *Basic Safety Rules:* 1) Place bands over clothing whenever possible to avoid pinching or rubbing skin and pulling body hair. 2) Look away from the band (especially in upper body strengthening) in the event it might break. 3) Do not use if you have high blood pressure, varicose veins, or are pregnant, due to increased blood pressure.
Surgical tubing:	Similar to rubber bands, but because tubing is open ended can have greater application in upper body work. Tubing can be tied to simulate rubber bands. Can be purchased at most medical supply stores for a few cents/foot and there are various thicknesses for progression of strengthening. Three to four foot lengths are necessary for each person. *Basic Safety Rules:* 1) Try not to snap but slowly lengthen. 2) Make sure you have a strong grip on both ends to prevent hitting yourself or another. If hands get tired, stop and rest.
Frisbees and Hula-hoops:	Make a different kind of warm up than stepping or moving in place. *Basic Safety Rules:* 1) More area is necessary. Keep activity "light" until stretching takes place. Use sponge frisbees for indoor areas. You may have to teach people how to throw a frisbee or use a hula-hoop correctly.

■ PORTABLE STRENGTHENING EQUIPMENT (CON'T)

Dowels or Canes:
For use as a prop with show tunes and dance routines. Three quarter to one inch dowels are the best.
Basic Safety Rules:
1) Need clearance on sides and overhead of each person. Position people with lots of room between them.

Balls:
From soft spongy balls (Nerf®) to red rubber playground balls, these can be used for range of motion movements, strengthening through a small range of movement by squeezing between body parts, used as a prop with regular exercises for variety and challenge (i.e., holding ball at arms length while performing curl-ups), for sports skills drills (ball handling like dribbling, figure 8 around the legs) and childhood games (1,2,3 O-Lario or passing over/under).
Basic Safety Rules:
1) For inflatable balls, underinflation helps people hold on or compress the ball without straining, but still allows the ball to bounce.
2) No throwing the ball at anyone without their permission, attention, and readiness (No bombardment here!).

Dumbbells or Hand weights:
Can be purchased or created with recycled materials donated by class members — tennis ball cans filled with sand (tape ends with duct or strapping tape); Soup cans (condensed soup works best); Plastic milk or juice containers marked with gradations for poundage, can be filled with sand or water (one gallon of water equals about 8 pounds).
Basic Safety Rules:
1) Care should be taken when lifting weight overhead — if you should lose a handhold — do not try to catch weight, but let it drop to the floor.
2) Always use proper body mechanics to pick up and put down weights. Use legs for lifting, keep weights close to body, use front to back stance — especially for lifting overhead and maintaining curves of spine.

Ankle weights:
Usually secured with straps or velcro.
Basic Safety Rules:
1) Use only with floor work, will throw off walking or running patterns.
2) Remind person wearing weights that number of repetitions will be reduced.
3) In exercises that use a straight leg (side leg lifts) person may have to return to bent knee lifts as weight has been added to the end of the lever arm.
4) Use controlled movements with lift *and* unlift. Benefit is gained returning weight to floor, do not just let weight and leg drop in response to gravity.

■ PORTABLE STRENGTHENING EQUIPMENT (CON'T)

Ropes: Can be used as an added prop for stretching, range of motion, resistance work, and aerobic activity. When used for resistance work, person supplies workload by pulling on ends of rope. If used for aerobic exercise, rope needs to be correct length for jumping (with person standing in middle of rope, ends should come up to armpit level on both sides).
Basic Safety Rules:
1) People need both horizontal and overhead clearance to swing rope for range of motion or effective jumping. Position people with 5-6 feet between them and 4-5 feet overhead.

Towels: Have each person bring a towel. Can be used as added prop for stretching, range of motion, and some resistance work can be accomplished with person or partner providing resistance.
Basic Safety Rules:
1) No snapping towels at anyone.
2) If partner is providing resistance, he/she needs to communicate with participant to establish the workload. Partner should not be applying so much resistance that participant cannot move smoothly through a range of motion.

Other instructors we know have used tennis balls, bean bags, and regular sponges for hand and forearm work. You also may have come up with different uses of everyday "stuff" to use in your classes. Although fancy equipment is great, most of us work in programs that do not budget for large quantities of equipment, nor do we have lots of storage space. In the examples above we have cited use of recycled materials. Not only is recycling good for the environment, but when people contribute to the class with materials, they step over the line from participant to contributor. Contribution adds another dimension to the exercise class, as members feel a stewardship toward themselves and their class.

As always, safety comes first— you may have thought that our mention of basic rules was obvious, but we have found from experience that with the use of props (especially balls), adults who should know better do things that a child might do — like throwing the ball at someone's face. Many times these actions are unintentional, but people do get hurt while "messing around." Anytime you use a prop or equipment, be sure to mention any safety precautions that might be necessary.

We have also found that while ankle and hand weights can be used during every class, other props are best if used periodically for variety, entertainment, and challenge. Other types of equipment that might combine aspects of both aerobic and strengthening work are circuit activities.

Cards or instruction for circuits and fitness activities need to be in place before the class actually gets underway so they can be introduced during the warm-up segment of the class. We recommend that when providing a circuit or fitness activity, that the majority of the exercises you select should be ones that you have used previously. Unless the circuit is to be used over a period of time and can be left in place, you don't have a great deal of time to introduce a totally new exercise plan. Introduce a few new exercises.

Circuit cards are easy to make, although they do take time. Directions should be short and easy to follow. A picture should be included, as well as options for the number of repetitions. Some examples of circuit cards follow.

■ CIRCUIT CARD EXAMPLES

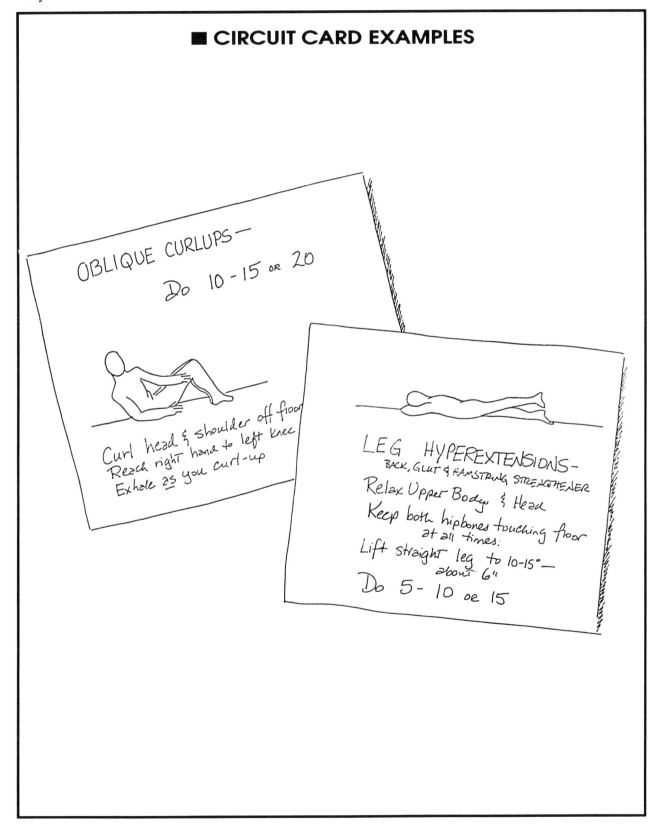

OBLIQUE CURLUPS —
Do 10 - 15 or 20

Curl head & shoulder off floor
Reach right hand to left knee
Exhale as you curl-up

LEG HYPEREXTENSIONS -
BACK, GLUT & HAMSTRING STRENGTHENER
Relax Upper Body & Head
Keep both hipbones touching floor
at all times.
Lift straight leg to 10-15° —
about 6"
Do 5 - 10 or 15

RELAXATION/ENERGIZE IS EMPHASIZED

■   During your class, people have been working hard, increasing the blood flow of nutrients and oxygen to the exercising muscles. Stiffness and muscular tension are now gone. As each minute of the class progresses, they let go of anxieties, worries, and stressors of the day. While the music was playing and they were moving to the beat, their brains switched from the logical and calculating functions and began operating on spontaneity, with fluid thought. Many ideas come, but no one idea or concern stays in focus as they walk, step, kick, push-up, bend and stretch. Many are pressed, too stressed, they had already made too many contacts with too many people — but they came anyway. That was the hardest part — coming to exercise class, and now they are glad they came. Their mindset is different now. They have taken the time to care for themselves. They have taken another step towards healthier living.

Now is the time for you to help your participants complete their journey. Take the last five minutes of your class to let your participants experience a few moments of increased relaxation or to re-energize before returning to their duties and commitments. These relaxation moments can be structured or free-flowing, philosophical, or quiet.

Silence or quiet, slow music (60 beats per minute or less) might be enough. Storytelling, guided imagery or creative visualization might help deepen the sensation as you describe quiet forests, gentle breezes, a warm fire, or a cozy room. Starbursts, bright, intense sunlight, the power of a wave or waterfall might suggest the energy necessary to continue on with the day's activities. Partner massage or group stories, deep breathing or progressively tightening and releasing muscle groups may help your participants find any remaining tensions, areas of pain, or resistance to change.

While your "audience" is receptive, you might use the time to compliment them on their hard work and reinforce their positive lifestyles, or help them perform a mental exercise to increase their self-esteem and personal power. You might read inspirational quotations or poetry or make annoucements about up-coming events. Whatever you might do — and by all means do what is comfortable for you, use these last few minutes to end the exercise experience on a positive note and allow participants to take their encounter past the allotted time.

In Chapter 9 we will take the extensive information on major muscle groups and movement just reviewed and use them to determine safe and effective exercise. Application of the SEARCH exercise analysis tool will allow you to look at muscle strengthening/endurance and stretching exercises to determine the best parts of each exercise, as well as give you cues on what needs to be changed or adapted.

REFERENCES

1. Blessing, D., Wilson, Puckett, J., and Ford, H. 1987. The Physiologic Effects of 8 Weeks of A.D. with and without hand-held weights. *American Journal of Sports Medicine* 15:5, 508-510.

2. Thompson, C. and Wells, C. Oct. 1989. CV Changes Associated with Low-impact Aerobic Dance with Light or Wrist Weights. Paper presented at International Symposium on the Scientific and Medical Aspects of Aerobic Dance Exercise, San Diego, CA.

SEARCH

FOR EXERCISE CHOICES

See in new ways _____

Explore the possibilities _____

Analyze the exercise _____

Right exercise for the right person _____

Choose effective _____

Healthy, lifetime exercise _____

Chapter 9

APPLICATION OF THE SEARCH EXERCISE ANALYSIS TOOL

A glance at most womens' magazines reveals that there is always a new, improved exercise program. This approach sells magazines. It also presents the same old stuff wrapped up in new packages. New packages are nice because they break up boredom and meet our need for novel and different ideas. Although if you have been teaching or exercising for any length of time, you have come to realize that the movements of the human body are finite or fixed with slight differences due to physical variation. When all of the packaging is stripped away, what do we really have? Does this exercise actually do anything, or is it just glitz, entertainment, or tradition? Does it DO what I think it does? Is this the best possible way to work this area of my body? Can I get hurt doing this exercise or activity?

Besides answering these questions concerning purpose and safety, we have come to realize that the most difficult thing to do while EXERCISING is TEACHING a group and MODIFYING exercise for the specific needs of the participant. What kinds of exercise would benefit my participants in their daily routines, recreational pursuits, and jobs? The ability to modify and individualize is necessary to turn the non-exerciser or sporadic exerciser into a regular participant. Some instructors can modify and individualize quickly and well, but we believe that if questioned, they would tell you that it takes practice and years of experience.

We would like to help you gain the ability to do this with the hope of circumventing some practice time. We believe that SEARCH can assist you in doing this; however you will still need to practice to make the technique your own.

In Chapter 7 we introduced SEARCH to get you to try analyzing exercises the way we do. We want you to think about how a particular exercise will fit into the total scheme of things. Chapter 8 reviewed the anatomy and function of the major muscle groups, exercises that need to be approached cautiously, and recommended exercises. We would now like to apply all of this useful information to practical situations. Sixteen exercises have been selected for analysis. Each page will show a picture of the exercise under scrutiny in conjunction with an actual SEARCH analysis. The worksheet comments describe how the exercise can be modified for better safety or more general use as well as a picture of the "finished product." We want you to experience the actual thought process that goes on whenever we discover or rediscover a "new" exercise; and how we go about "testing" an exercise before putting it into use. These thoughts are ours, however. As you read our comments, you might have something to add or argue. These remarks are a matter of judgment and experience. They are the gray areas of exercise. This "mental sparring" helps prepare you for the "mental jogging" that becomes necessary when leading a class.

We would like to reassure you that the analysis eventually becomes second nature. After seeing a new exercise you will automatically begin to analyze it by selecting the good parts and modifying the rest. We only wish that we could share this process with you in person. Input and questions from instructors at workshops inspired the idea to create SEARCH and this entire book.

Before you begin reading the analyses, a quick review of the SEARCH tool might be helpful. If you remember Chapter 7's introduction, the best score an exercise could receive would be six YES answers. Any variation from this score would cause you to:

A. pinpoint the problem areas.
B. modify the aspects of an exercise that would increase the number of YES answers.
C. evaluate any aspect that could not be modified.

If the risk to benefit ratio is too high, it would be much wiser to choose another alternative. Look quickly at the complete SEARCH tool again before proceeding to the following analyses.

■ SEARCH EXERCISE ANALYSIS TOOL

DETERMINE IF THE OVERALL PURPOSE OF THE EXERCISE IS TO IMPROVE FLEXIBILITY OR MUSCLE STRENGTH AND ENDURANCE.

Complete the section below, checking the appropriate boxes under "Yes," "Maybe," or "No."

FLEXIBILITY	Yes	Maybe	No
A. Is it important to perform this exercise to counteract the effects of activities of daily life, work, and/or to prepare for recreational pursuits?	( )	( )	( )
B. Is the exercise shown and cued in a biomechanically correct way, with possible modifications presented?	( )	( )	( )
C. Is there adequate base of support?	( )	( )	( )
D. Does the stretch allow for maximum muscle relaxation and minimization of gravitational pull?	( )	( )	( )
E. Is this exercise performed using controlled, non-ballistic movements?	( )	( )	( )
F. Can this exercise be performed *without* compromising other body parts?	( )	( )	( )

MUSCLE STRENGTH AND ENDURANCE	Yes	Maybe	No
A. Is it important to perform this exercise to counteract the effects of activities of daily life, work, and/or to prepare for recreational pursuits?	( )	( )	( )
B. Is the exercise shown and cued in a biomechanically correct way, with possible modifications presented?	( )	( )	( )
C. Is there adequate base of support?	( )	( )	( )
D. Does the exercise work the muscle(s) through the full and correct joint range of motion?	( )	( )	( )
E. Is this exercise performed using controlled, isotonic, non-ballistic movements?	( )	( )	( )
F. Can this exercise be performed *without* compromising other body parts?	( )	( )	( )

■ SEARCH EXERCISE ANALYSIS TOOL
Small Arm Circles

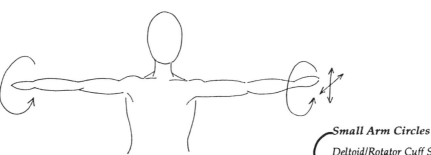

Small Arm Circles

Deltoid/Rotator Cuff Strengthening more like "Entertainment"

SEARCH for Exercise Choices Worksheet

DETERMINE IF THE OVERALL PURPOSE OF THE EXERCISE IS TO IMPROVE FLEXIBILITY OR MUSCLE STRENGTH AND ENDURANCE

Complete the section below, checking the appropriate boxes under "Yes," "Maybe," or "No."

MUSCLE STRENGTH AND ENDURANCE

	Yes	Maybe	No
A. Is it important to perform this exercise to counteract the effects of activities of daily life, work, and/or to prepare for recreational pursuits?	( )	( )	☒
B. Is the exercise shown and cued in a biomechanically correct way, with possible modifications presented?	( )	( )	☒
C. Is there adequate base of support?	( )	( )	☒
D. Does the exercise work the muscle(s) through the full and correct joint range of motion?	( )	( )	☒
E. Is this exercise performed using controlled, isotonic, non-ballistic movements?	( )	( )	☒
F. Can this exercise be performed *without* compromising other body parts?	( )	( )	☒

A. *Do you carry anything this way? Do you perform any work activities this way? These movements are often overdone and are more entertainment, although not completely safe . . . read on.*

C. *The base of support ends up being the shoulder joint, muscles of the rotator cuff, and the deltoids. In this position muscles of the rotator cuff are maximally contracted.*

D. *Muscles are not worked through the full range of motion.*

E. *Movements are very ballistic, shortened, and become very isometric. Lack of blood flow is what causes pain and discomfort.*

F. *Will likely compromise shoulder joint, rotator cuff muscles, and elevate blood pressure.*

Need for Modification — Cuing Tips

1) *Need to increase range of motion.*

2) *Use of different angles and planes to decrease stress on deltoids and rotator cuff.*

3) *Avoid quick, short, choppy movements.*

4) *Bend elbows at times while working through different angles and planes.*

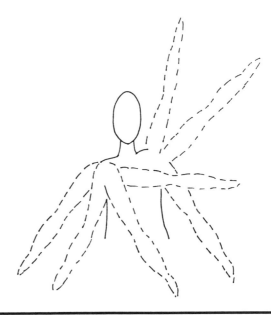

■ SEARCH EXERCISE ANALYSIS TOOL
Abdominal Compressions

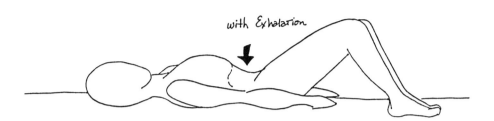

with Exhalation

Abdominal Compressions

Abdominal Strengthening

SEARCH for Exercise Choices Worksheet

DETERMINE IF THE OVERALL PURPOSE OF THE EXERCISE IS TO IMPROVE FLEXIBILITY OR MUSCLE STRENGTH AND ENDURANCE

Complete the section below, checking the appropriate boxes under "Yes," "Maybe," or "No."

MUSCLE STRENGTH AND ENDURANCE

		Yes	Maybe	No
A.	*It is important to strengthen abdominals this way because this is what is needed for posture, body mechanics, particularly lifting.* A. Is it important to perform this exercise to counteract the effects of activities of daily life, work, and/or to prepare for recreational pursuits?	☒	( )	( )
D.	*Can work through the full range of motion since the compressive action is different than flexion.* B. Is the exercise shown and cued in a biomechanically correct way, with possible modifications presented?	☒	( )	( )
E.	*Good for warming up diaphragm before exercise, and for deep breathing during relaxation.* C. Is there adequate base of support?	☒	( )	( )
F.	*Could elevate blood pressure if breath is held. Exhaling with compressions simulates what people need to do with lifting — pull abdominals into splint and stabilize lumbar spine.* D. Does the exercise work the muscle(s) through the full and correct joint range of motion?	( )	☒	( )
	E. Is this exercise performed using controlled, isotonic, non-ballistic movements?	☒	( )	( )
	F. Can this exercise be performed *without* compromising other body parts?	☒	( )	( )

Need for Modification — Cuing Tips

1) *No modifications needed - a good exercise for almost everyone.*

2) *Inhale - when your body needs to exhale - begin breathing out, pulling abdominals in as tight as possible. Let need to inhale initiate release of the compression.*

3) *The reason to couple this exercise with smooth, deep breathing is to prevent sudden compression, which could initiate a back spasm or could increase back pain; increase breathing and exercise diaphragm (you are doing diaphragmmatic breathing here; an important technique for exercise); allow for relaxed breathing, an essential of all relaxation techniques.*

4) *Relate to posture and lifting technique as in F.*

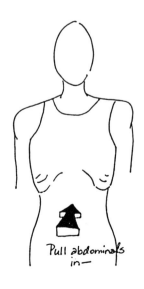

Pull abdominals in—

■ SEARCH EXERCISE ANALYSIS TOOL
Wall Sits

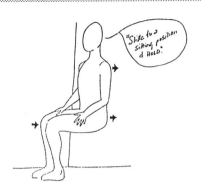

Wall Sits

Quadriceps strengthening

SEARCH for Exercise Choices Worksheet

DETERMINE IF THE OVERALL PURPOSE OF THE EXERCISE IS TO IMPROVE FLEXIBILITY OR MUSCLE STRENGTH AND ENDURANCE

Complete the section below, checking the appropriate boxes under "Yes," "Maybe," or "No."

MUSCLE STRENGTH AND ENDURANCE

	Yes	Maybe	No
A. Is it important to perform this exercise to counteract the effects of activities of daily life, work, and/or to prepare for recreational pursuits?	( )	( )	☒
B. Is the exercise shown and cued in a biomechanically correct way, with possible modifications presented?	( )	( )	☒
C. Is there adequate base of support?	☒	( )	( )
D. Does the exercise work the muscle(s) through the full and correct joint range of motion?	( )	( )	☒
E. Is this exercise performed using controlled, isotonic, non-ballistic movements?	( )	( )	☒
F. Can this exercise be performed *without* compromising other body parts?	( )	( )	☒

A. *No, because it strengthens a limited range of motion. Even with sports activities requiring jumping or bent knee positions there are better alternatives.*

B. *As presented, come to a sitting position and hold - no modifications given.*

C. *If weight is pressed against the wall, feet out approximately 2 feet from the wall.*

D. *No, not at all. Strengthens a very limited range of motion.*

E. *There is no movement, especially isotonic movement. This exercise is highly isometric.*

F. *This position puts a great deal of compressive force on the knee joints. Because of the isometric nature of this exercise, elevations of blood pressure are common. Do not use for individuals with blood pressure problems.*

Need for Modification — Cuing Tips

1) *Changing the static position to dynamic movement will make this exercise isotonic, strengthening through an expanded range of motion, without elevating the blood pressure and straining the knee joints.*

2) *Wall sliding instead of wall sitting is a good transition exercise for strengthening the quadriceps with partial weight bearing. This is a good way for injured people to strengthen and progress to full weight bearing away from the wall.*

3) *Remind people: "Slide down the wall to the point where you are able to reverse directions and come back to the standing position. Do not allow yourself to get stuck in a sitting position."*

"You do not want to train your muscles in a sitting position since a backward sitting position is not used for any activity except falling backward (not good on the ski slope)."

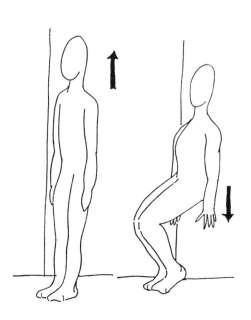

■ SEARCH EXERCISE ANALYSIS TOOL
Outer Thigh Strengthening

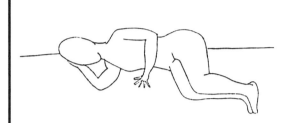 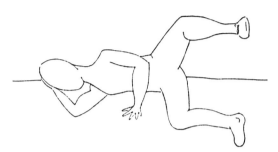

Outer Thigh Strengthening

SEARCH for Exercise Choices Worksheet

DETERMINE IF THE OVERALL PURPOSE OF THE EXERCISE IS TO IMPROVE FLEXIBILITY OR MUSCLE STRENGTH AND ENDURANCE

Complete the section below, checking the appropriate boxes under "Yes," "Maybe," or "No."

MUSCLE STRENGTH AND ENDURANCE

		Yes	Maybe	No
A.	Is it important to perform this exercise to counteract the effects of activities of daily life, work, and/or to prepare for recreational pursuits?	( )	( )	☒
B.	Is the exercise shown and cued in a biomechanically correct way, with possible modifications presented?	☒	( )	( )
C.	Is there adequate base of support?	☒	( )	( )
D.	Does the exercise work the muscle(s) through the full and correct joint range of motion?	(☒	( )	( )
E.	Is this exercise performed using controlled, isotonic, non-ballistic movements?	☒	( )	( )
F.	Can this exercise be performed *without* compromising other body parts?	( )	☒	( )

A. *These types of exercises work the gluteus medius, which is a small muscle that is strong enough from daily activities. Most people believe this will help them shape up their hips and instructors using many of these are promoting spot reducing.*

C. *Bent knee and arm in front will stabilize base of support. The bent knee (vs. using a straight leg) decreases the weight of the lift by decreasing the leverage.*

D. *Allows for abduction of 45°.*

F. *This position can increase pressure in the hip capsule and also isolates the gluteus medius almost too much! The gluteus medius is a small muscle — use less repetitions in this position.*

Need for Modification

1) *Rotating the hip medially will work the gluteus effectively.*

2) *Safe exercise for most people.*

3) *Avoid using this exercise a great deal to avoid excessive pressure on the hip joint and to avoid giving the message that "spot reducing" is possible.*

Cuing Tips

4) *Relax head on arm.*

5) *Bend hips and knees at 90° — like you would if you were sitting on a chair.*

6) *Place your left hand on floor in front of you to stabilize your base.*

7) *Lift smoothly to 45°.*

■ SEARCH EXERCISE ANALYSIS TOOL
Knee Bends

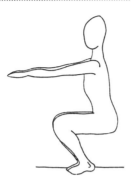

SEARCH for Exercise Choices Worksheet

Knee Bends
Quadriceps strengthening

DETERMINE IF THE OVERALL PURPOSE OF THE EXERCISE IS TO IMPROVE FLEXIBILITY OR MUSCLE STRENGTH AND ENDURANCE

Complete the section below, checking the appropriate boxes under "Yes," "Maybe," or "No."

MUSCLE STRENGTH AND ENDURANCE

		Yes	Maybe	No
A.	Is it important to perform this exercise to counteract the effects of activities of daily life, work, and/or to prepare for recreational pursuits?	☒	( )	( )
B.	Is the exercise shown and cued in a biomechanically correct way, with possible modifications presented?	☒	( )	( )
C.	Is there adequate base of support?	( )	( )	☒
D.	Does the exercise work the muscle(s) through the full and correct joint range of motion?	( )	( )	☒
E.	Is this exercise performed using controlled, isotonic, non-ballistic movements?	( )	☒	( )
F.	Can this exercise be performed *without* compromising other body parts?	( )	☒	( )

A. Yes, it is important to have strong legs for daily lifting tasks, and application of correct body mechanics.

B. As presented, the exercise shows using the arms as a counterbalance, keeping the thigh parallel to the floor (avoiding "deep" knee bends), and use of good posture.

C. Even with heels flat, many people cannot perform this exercise without losing their balance because most of the body weight is in the back.

D/F. "Deep" knee bends greatly stress the structures of the knee, but are often necessary for correct lifting technique. Shortening the range of motion does not prepare the body as well for lifting, but does save the knees while strengthening the quadriceps.

E. The arms are held in isometric position. The legs may also end up in isometric contraction if the position is held.

Need for Modification — Cuing Tips

1) Knee protection is particularly necessary if the participant does this a great deal in daily activities. Encourage all participants to use this posture and these techniques in daily activities and when picking up objects in class. Make sure you demonstrate and use this position as well.

2) Increase the base of support by taking a front to back stance. This stance can also be widened from side to side.

3) Avoid isometrics that occur with holding the squatted position, or bouncing at the bottom of the squat by using smooth, slow and controlled movements. Bring arms up smoothly to counterbalance at the deepest part of the squat. Bring arms down as legs straighten.

4) Talk posture! Chin up! Maintain the curves of the spine.

5) Instruct participants with knee problems to bend knees only as far as comfortable, go no further than "comfort zone."

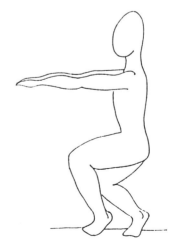

■ SEARCH EXERCISE ANALYSIS TOOL
Abdominal Strengthening

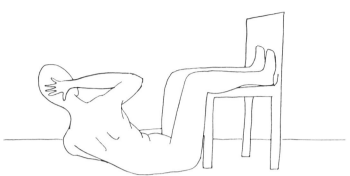

Abdominal Strengthening

SEARCH for Exercise Choices Worksheet

DETERMINE IF THE OVERALL PURPOSE OF THE EXERCISE IS TO IMPROVE FLEXIBILITY OR MUSCLE STRENGTH AND ENDURANCE

Complete the section below, checking the appropriate boxes under "Yes," "Maybe," or "No."

MUSCLE STRENGTH AND ENDURANCE

		Yes	Maybe	No
A.	Is it important to perform this exercise to counteract the effects of activities of daily life, work, and/or to prepare for recreational pursuits?	☒	( )	( )
B.	Is the exercise shown and cued in a biomechanically correct way, with possible modifications presented?	☒	( )	( )
C.	Is there adequate base of support?	☒	( )	( )
D.	Does the exercise work the muscle(s) through the full and correct joint range of motion?	☒	( )	( )
E.	Is this exercise performed using controlled, isotonic, non-ballistic movements?	☒	( )	( )
F.	Can this exercise be performed *without* compromising other body parts?	( )	☒	( )

A. *Abdominal strengthening is important for back support. The exercise presents oblique work, which is also important – since the obliques wrap around the torso and are part of the muscular unit of the back.*

B./D. *The hips are at 90° with legs supported by the chair. This position helps to isolate the abdominals and minimizes use of the iliopsoas muscle group.*

C. *With the left shoulder on the ground, the upper back/shoulder muscles remain relaxed. Isolation of the oblique muscles occurs while the base of support is very stable.*

F. *The neck muscles may get fatigued before the abdominal muscles, needing the support presented. Some individuals with back problems may have difficulty with the element of twisting, although some twisting is essential in daily living.*

Need for Modification — Cuing

1) *This exercise needs little, if any, modification and would be a good exercise for almost anyone.*

2) *Getting into and out of position could be a problem for some individuals.*

   •*Roll on side, get hips as close to chair as possible, roll onto back, bringing legs up to the seat of the chair. To get up after exercise is completed – roll onto side, push up to hands and knees, stand.*

3) *Curl head followed by shoulder toward opposite knee. Concentrate on pointing shoulder to opposite knee, not elbow.*

4) *To avoid any compromise of neck structures, avoid pulling head forcefully and relax head in hand. Decrease range initially for low back problems.*

5) *Take deep breath in before lifting head, exhale as you curl up.*

■ SEARCH EXERCISE ANALYSIS TOOL
Full Sit-ups

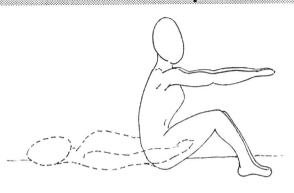

Full Sit-ups
Abdominal Strengthening

SEARCH for Exercise Choices Worksheet

DETERMINE IF THE OVERALL PURPOSE OF THE EXERCISE IS TO IMPROVE FLEXIBILITY OR MUSCLE STRENGTH AND ENDURANCE

Complete the section below, checking the appropriate boxes under "Yes," "Maybe," or "No."

MUSCLE STRENGTH AND ENDURANCE

		Yes	Maybe	No
A.	Is it important to perform this exercise to counteract the effects of activities of daily life, work, and/or to prepare for recreational pursuits?	( )	(X)	( )
B.	Is the exercise shown and cued in a biomechanically correct way, with possible modifications presented?	( )	( )	(X)
C.	Is there adequate base of support?	(X)	( )	( )
D.	Does the exercise work the muscle(s) through the full and correct joint range of motion?	( )	(X)	( )
E.	Is this exercise performed using controlled, isotonic, non-ballistic movements?	( )	(X)	( )
F.	Can this exercise be performed *without* compromising other body parts?	( )	(X)	( )

A. *While it is important to strengthen the abdominal muscles, it is also important to consider that we do a great deal of forward flexion daily.*

B. *The picture shows the sit-up, but not the phase returning to the floor. The return to the floor is the phase where back strain can occur. Support for the neck also needs to be considered.*

D. *The exercise as presented does go through the range of motion and beyond 80° where the hip flexors finish the movement.*

E. *People performing full sit-ups often use the arms and snapping motion of the pelvis to supply the momentum to sit-up, rather than using the abdominal muscles.*

F. *The exerciser might injure his/her back unless he/she rolls up and rolls down with each repetition.*

Need for Modification — Cuing

1) *Since flexion is not needed and even discouraged in activities of daily living, curl-up instead of sitting up, and emphasize compressions and obliques.*

2) *Avoid compromise of low back by:*

   • *Keep low back flat on the floor by having knees bent and pressing back flat against the floor.*
   • *Curl head and shoulders until shoulder blades barely lift off the floor.*
   • *Roll up touching each vertebrae; roll down the same way.*

3) *Avoid compromise of neck by:*

   • *Relaxing your head in your hands.*
   • *Look at your knees, avoid crunching your head toward your chest.*

4) *Exhale as you curl up, inhale while rolling down.*

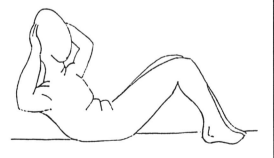

■ SEARCH EXERCISE ANALYSIS TOOL
Back Strengthening

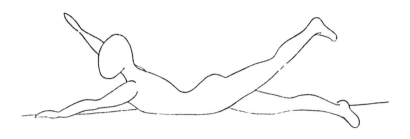

Back Strengthening

SEARCH for Exercise Choices Worksheet

DETERMINE IF THE OVERALL PURPOSE OF THE EXERCISE IS TO IMPROVE FLEXIBILITY OR MUSCLE STRENGTH AND ENDURANCE

Complete the section below, checking the appropriate boxes under "Yes," "Maybe," or "No."

MUSCLE STRENGTH AND ENDURANCE

A. *We do need to counteract all of the effects of flexion in daily activities. Hyperextension does strengthen the back.*

B. *As presented – looks very difficult, requires coordination.*

C. *One hand, abdomen, leg opposite is base of support.*

D. *Leg lift is beyond range of motion.*

E. *As presented – looks difficult to control, movements would have a tendency to become ballistic with changes from side to side.*

F. *Compromises low back. Holding breath during movements might elevate blood pressure.*

	Yes	Maybe	No
A. Is it important to perform this exercise to counteract the effects of activities of daily life, work, and/or to prepare for recreational pursuits?	☒	( )	( )
B. Is the exercise shown and cued in a biomechanically correct way, with possible modifications presented?	( )	( )	☒
C. Is there adequate base of support?	( )	☒	( )
D. Does the exercise work the muscle(s) through the full and correct joint range of motion?	( )	( )	☒
E. Is this exercise performed using controlled, isotonic, non-ballistic movements?	( )	☒	( )
F. Can this exercise be performed *without* compromising other body parts?	( )	( )	☒

Need for Modification

1) *Keep hipbones on ground at all times to decrease leg lifts to correct range of motion.*

2) *Head, arm, and leg lift all at the same time, may compromise the low back – keep head down and arm in line with head. Keep non-lifted arm in contact with ground to help increase base of support.*

3) *Avoid uncontrolled, ballistic movements – lift smoothly, slowly and carefully.*

4) *Instruct people to breathe "with the work" or when lifting.*

5) *Should only be used after a progression or series can be performed without difficulty (i.e. raise one arm at a time; raise one leg at a time; no problems – then present this challenge!).*

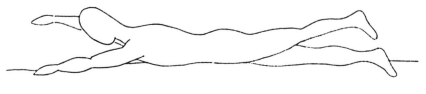

■ SEARCH EXERCISE ANALYSIS TOOL
Hamstring/Gluteal Strengthening

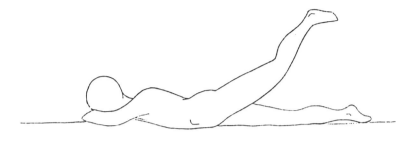

Hamstring/Gluteal
Strengthening

SEARCH for Exercise Choices Worksheet

DETERMINE IF THE OVERALL PURPOSE OF THE EXERCISE IS TO IMPROVE FLEXIBILITY OR MUSCLE STRENGTH AND ENDURANCE

Complete the section below, checking the appropriate boxes under "Yes," "Maybe," or "No."

MUSCLE STRENGTH AND ENDURANCE

A. *Hamstrings do need strengthening and activities for strengthening without equipment are limited.*

B. *Goes beyond suggested range of motion (10-15°), which may put excessive pressure on intervertebral discs and back muscles.*

D. *Is beyond full and correct range of motion – as above. In order to lift leg this high, hipbone must be off of floor.*

E. *This would be one exercise that could be easily performed ballistically or if head at top of lift, would be very isometric. Isometrics could elevate blood pressure.*

F. *As shown, would compromise low back as mentioned in B, but raising leg off of floor with hipbone off of floor as well, results in lifting and twisting — a surefire way to get injured.*

	Yes	Maybe	No
A. Is it important to perform this exercise to counteract the effects of activities of daily life, work, and/or to prepare for recreational pursuits?	☒	( )	( )
B. Is the exercise shown and cued in a biomechanically correct way, with possible modifications presented?	( )	( )	☒
C. Is there adequate base of support?	☒	( )	( )
D. Does the exercise work the muscle(s) through the full and correct joint range of motion?	( )	( )	☒
E. Is this exercise performed using controlled, isotonic, non-ballistic movements?	( )	☒	( )
F. Can this exercise be performed *without* compromising other body parts?	( )	☒	( )

Need for Modification - Cuing Tips

1) *Keep hipbones on floor at all times.*

2) *Lift your leg with your knee locked about 10-15 ° — 6-12 inches.*

3) *Inhale - then exhale as you lift the leg smoothly. Avoid holding your breath.*

4) *Even with modifications this may be difficult or contraindicated in some participants with back problems.*

■ SEARCH EXERCISE ANALYSIS TOOL
Full Push-ups

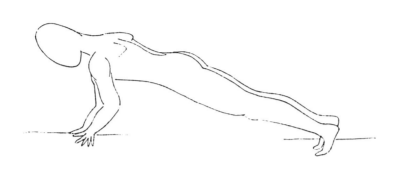

Full Push-ups

*Pectorals/Bicep/Upper Back
Strengthening*

SEARCH for Exercise Choices Worksheet

DETERMINE IF THE OVERALL PURPOSE OF THE EXERCISE IS TO IMPROVE FLEXIBILITY OR MUSCLE STRENGTH AND ENDURANCE

Complete the section below, checking the appropriate boxes under "Yes," "Maybe," or "No."

A. *Chest muscles are generally tight enough because most work and daily activities are performed in the front of the body. Some individuals may need to increase or maintain upper body strength because of lifting requirements for work or daily living.*

B. *Many people cannot perform this exercise without modification – for example, a change in hand position or decrease in body weight.*

C. *The only base is the hands and toes, supporting the full body weight of the individual. This exercise may also be quite difficult if exerciser does not have a broad shoulder girdle.*

D. *This exercise could work the muscles through the full range of motion if the person is strong enough to perform the lift and maintain rigid body position.*

F. *May compromise wrists, shoulders, elbows, forearms and/or lower back if person is unable to maintain rigid position, or these structures are not strong enough to lift the body weight.*

MUSCLE STRENGTH AND ENDURANCE

	Yes	Maybe	No
A. Is it important to perform this exercise to counteract the effects of activities of daily life, work, and/or to prepare for recreational pursuits?	( )	☒	( )
B. Is the exercise shown and cued in a biomechanically correct way, with possible modifications presented?	( )	☒	( )
C. Is there adequate base of support?	( )	( )	☒
D. Does the exercise work the muscle(s) through the full and correct joint range of motion?	( )	☒	( )
E. Is this exercise performed using controlled, isotonic, non-ballistic movements?	☒	( )	( )
F. Can this exercise be performed *without* compromising other body parts?	( )	( )	☒

Need for Modification - Cuing Tips

1) *Increase base of support by keeping knees and lower legs in contact with ground (knee push-ups).*

2) *Increasing the base of support also decreases body weight, changes leverage and does not require as much rigidity of the torso, which may decrease compromise of upper extremity structures and the back.*

3) *Work up to lifting full body weight by adding body weight in increments (first wall push-ups, to upper body press-ups, to knee push-ups, to full push-ups).*

4) *People with narrow shoulder girdle may need wider hand width.*

5) *Wall push-ups are best for participants with knee, hand and wrist problems.*

6) *Perform push-ups before abdominal exercises since it is harder to maintain torso rigidity.*

7) *Emphasize breathing technique – exhale with lowering body to floor (this requires control); inhale with lift. Helps support low back.*

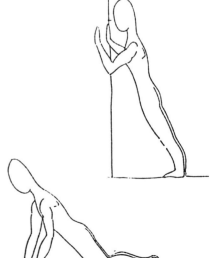

■ SEARCH EXERCISE ANALYSIS TOOL
Abdominal Strengthening

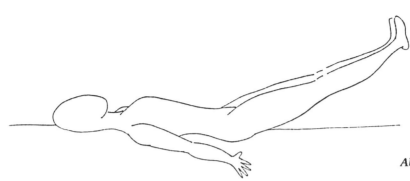

Abdominal Strengthener?

SEARCH for Exercise Choices Worksheet

DETERMINE IF THE OVERALL PURPOSE OF THE EXERCISE IS TO IMPROVE FLEXIBILITY OR MUSCLE STRENGTH AND ENDURANCE

Complete the section below, checking the appropriate boxes under "Yes," "Maybe," or "No."

MUSCLE STRENGTH AND ENDURANCE

		Yes	Maybe	No
A.	*It is important to strengthen abdominals — abdominals working by compression here, and that is important.*			
	A. Is it important to perform this exercise to counteract the effects of activities of daily life, work, and/or to prepare for recreational pursuits?	☒	( )	( )
B.	*This exercise is really working the deep muscles of the back and the iliopsoas — weight of legs extended, pulls directly on low back.*			
	B. Is the exercise shown and cued in a biomechanically correct way, with possible modifications presented?	( )	( )	☒
C.	*Head, back, and buttocks are the base of support, but with legs extended, a long, heavy lever is created, making the back unstable.*			
	C. Is there adequate base of support?	( )	☒	( )
D.	*As presented there is no range of motion for abdominals. There is slight range of motion for the iliopsoas muscles.*			
	D. Does the exercise work the muscle(s) through the full and correct joint range of motion?	( )	( )	☒
E.	*The movement appears controlled, however movement to this position might be ballistic in nature. This exercise is highly isometric for legs, abdominals, back muscles, and arms.*			
	E. Is this exercise performed using controlled, isotonic, non-ballistic movements?	( )	( )	☒
F.	*Often is presented as being acceptable if low back is maintained in a pelvic tilt. This is extremely difficult even for very strong individuals. Strong abdominal compression is needed to maintain/ stabilize low back — most individuals do not have this type of strength. May greatly elevate blood pressure.*			
	F. Can this exercise be performed *without* compromising other body parts?	( )	( )	☒

Need for Modification - Cuing Tips

1) *Works on abdominal compression and pelvic tilt which are needed, but there are better ways to accomplish these exercises that have no risk.*

2) *Could modify by keeping one knee bent and performing a straight leg raise, this however, does not strengthen abdominals - but quads/hip flexors - already plenty strong.*

3) *This is highly isometric — resulting in greatly elevated blood pressure, dangerous for some individuals.*

4) *High potential for back injury due to traction type pull on deep muscles of low back; weight of legs in this pull also adds to problem.*

Any modifications would result in a complete change of the exercise to better alternatives. Leaving as is— means high risk to benefit —use those better alternatives.

■ SEARCH EXERCISE ANALYSIS TOOL
Quadriceps/Hip Flexor Stretch

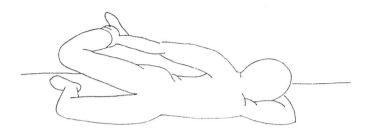

Quadriceps/Hip Flexor Stretch

SEARCH for Exercise Choices Worksheet

DETERMINE IF THE OVERALL PURPOSE OF THE EXERCISE IS TO IMPROVE FLEXIBILITY OR MUSCLE STRENGTH AND ENDURANCE

Complete the section below, checking the appropriate boxes under "Yes," "Maybe," or "No."

FLEXIBILITY

Yes Maybe No

A. Is it important to perform this exercise to counteract the effects of activities of daily life, work, and/or to prepare for recreational pursuits?   ☒ ( ) ( )

B. Is the exercise shown and cued in a biomechanically correct way, with possible modifications presented?   ☒ ( ) ( )

C. Is there adequate base of support?   ( ) ☒ ( )

D. Does the stretch allow for maximum muscle relaxation and minimization of gravitational pull?   ☒ ( ) ( )

E. Is this exercise performed using controlled, non-ballistic movements?   ☒ ( ) ( )

F. Can this exercise be performed *without* compromising other body parts?   ☒ ( ) ( )

A. *With a lot of daily sitting, most people have the need to stretch the quadriceps group and hip flexors.*

B. *Heel is not being pulled to buttocks, but is shown held in a relaxed, supportive position.*

C. *Bottom leg is bent to increase stability and base of support. Lying on the stomach would be the best base of support.*

E. *Appears to be relaxed and controlled stretch.*

F. *By not pulling heel toward buttock, the knee joint would not be compromised. Keeping head resting on arm would keep neck from being compromised.*

Need for Modification - Cuing Tips

1)   *No modifications needed — good exercise for almost anyone.*

2)   *Lie on side, one arm supporting head.*

3)   *Bend knee of leg closest to the floor to stabilize position, prevent twisting, or falling forward or backward.*

4)   *Foot does not have to touch buttocks for stretch to be effective.*

5)   *Leg should be relaxed by supporting with hand.*

6)   *Keep knees and hips in line.*

7)   *Find a comfortable stretch — then hold!*

■ SEARCH EXERCISE ANALYSIS TOOL
Hamstring Stretch

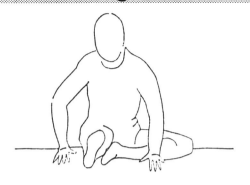

Hamstring Stretch

SEARCH for Exercise Choices Worksheet

DETERMINE IF THE OVERALL PURPOSE OF THE EXERCISE IS TO IMPROVE FLEXIBILITY OR MUSCLE STRENGTH AND ENDURANCE

Complete the section below, checking the appropriate boxes under "Yes," "Maybe," or "No."

FLEXIBILITY

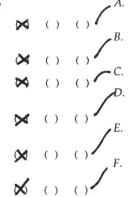

		Yes	Maybe	No	
A.	Is it important to perform this exercise to counteract the effects of activities of daily life, work, and/or to prepare for recreational pursuits?	☒	( )	( )	*A. Hamstring stretches important to counteract effects of sitting.*
B.	Is the exercise shown and cued in a biomechanically correct way, with possible modifications presented?	☒	( )	( )	*B. Appears presentation is good. Torso is erect. Head is up. Leg is straight out from hip.*
C.	Is there adequate base of support?	☒	( )	( )	*C. Bent knee might help stabilize base of support.*
D.	Does the stretch allow for maximum muscle relaxation and minimization of gravitational pull?	☒	( )	( )	*D. Hamstring group would be relaxed in this position—gravity minimized.*
E.	Is this exercise performed using controlled, non-ballistic movements?	☒	( )	( )	*E. Cue would need to stress going to comfortable position and hold.*
F.	Can this exercise be performed *without* compromising other body parts?	☒	( )	( )	*F. Uses arms to support torso—minimizes any compromise of back.*

Need for Modification - Cuing Tips

1) *Good choice for most exercisers, especially beginners, injured participants, mixed groups!*

■ SEARCH EXERCISE ANALYSIS TOOL
Hamstring Stretch

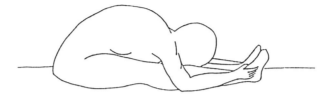

Hamstring Stretch

SEARCH for Exercise Choices Worksheet

DETERMINE IF THE OVERALL PURPOSE OF THE EXERCISE IS TO IMPROVE FLEXIBILITY OR MUSCLE STRENGTH AND ENDURANCE

Complete the section below, checking the appropriate boxes under "Yes," "Maybe," or "No."

FLEXIBILITY

Yes   Maybe   No

A. Is it important to perform this exercise to counteract the effects of activities of daily life, work, and/or to prepare for recreational pursuits?
( )   (X)   ( )

B. Is the exercise shown and cued in a biomechanically correct way, with possible modifications presented?
( )   ( )   (X)

C. Is there adequate base of support?
(X)   ( )   ( )

D. Does the stretch allow for maximum muscle relaxation and minimization of gravitational pull?
(X)   ( )   ( )

E. Is this exercise performed using controlled, non-ballistic movements?
( )   (X)   ( )

F. Can this exercise be performed *without* compromising other body parts?
( )   (X)   ( )

A. Good to stretch hamstrings, but this exercise also stretches the upper back, something we do too much of in everyday activities, and if we "slouch" with poor posture.

B. The back has lost its low back curve and therefore its ability to withstand compressive forces. The stretch, as presented, seems beyond the capabilities of most people.

E. Participants with decreased flexibility might bounce or overstretch to achieve this position.

F. May compromise the low back. When we try the stretch as presented, we feel more stretch in the upper and low back instead of the hamstrings. If a person sits up from this position, he/she would lift with back muscles and might get injured.

Need for Modification - Cuing Tips

1) *Maintain curve of spine by keeping head up. Staying erect and extended will maintain compressive capabilities of spine.*

2) *Keeping head up and aiming chin at feet will maximize the hamstring stretch.*

3) *"Walk" hands down legs until you find a comfortable stretch and hold. Keep hands in place to support low back.*

4) *"Walk" hands up legs to avoid using back to lift torso.*

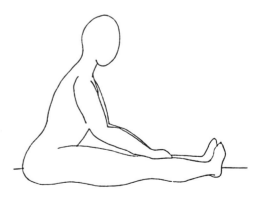

■ SEARCH EXERCISE ANALYSIS TOOL
The Yoga Plough

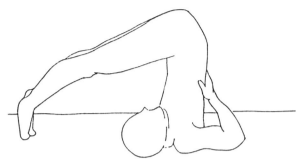

The Yoga Plough

Stretches hamstrings and low back

SEARCH for Exercise Choices Worksheet

DETERMINE IF THE OVERALL PURPOSE OF THE EXERCISE IS TO IMPROVE FLEXIBILITY OR MUSCLE STRENGTH AND ENDURANCE

Complete the section below, checking the appropriate boxes under "Yes," "Maybe," or "No."

FLEXIBILITY

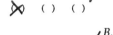

Yes Maybe No

A. Is it important to perform this exercise to counteract the effects of activities of daily life, work, and/or to prepare for recreational pursuits? ☒ ( ) ( )

B. Is the exercise shown and cued in a biomechanically correct way, with possible modifications presented? ( ) ( ) ☒

C. Is there adequate base of support? ( ) ( ) ☒

D. Does the stretch allow for maximum muscle relaxation and minimization of gravitational pull? ( ) ( ) ☒

E. Is this exercise performed using controlled, non-ballistic movements? ( ) ☒ ( )

F. Can this exercise be performed *without* compromising other body parts? ( ) ( ) ☒

A. Important to stretch low back and hamstrings to counter the effects of daily activities. Is an advanced exercise in yoga.

B. Appears to be an extreme position — for most people. No intermediate position presented.

C. Support toes, head, neck, shoulders, upper arms — not the best support for most of body weight.

D. Back is being held up against gravity, a lot of gravitational pull on legs — doesn't look or feel very relaxing when tried.

E. Need momentum to get into this position. Holding position in controlled, non-ballistic way would require flexibility and strength.

F. Appears to put a great deal of body weight (hips and legs) over cervical spine. Cervical spine is not built to support great amount of weight. Weight over neck makes breathing difficult. Extreme pull on back, hips, hamstrings, calves.

Need for Modification - Cuing Tips

1) *Please note: Even with modifications this exercise is not for everyone. We chose to show and analyze this exercise to illustrate how some exercises taken from other exercise systems should not be used generally, but only with selected groups or individuals (those individuals who demonstrate good range and flexibility in hamstrings and low back stretches, non-injured participants or athletes, or individuals participating in yoga instruction as part of a progression).*

2) *Since the exercise illustrated above compromises so much and has a risky base of support, increase the base by keeping the head and upper body on the floor. This increased base will also reduce the weight over the upper body, increase relaxation, and decrease the intensity of the stretch.*

3) *Cue people to -*

   *— Keep hips and legs over torso, **not** neck or upper body.*

   — Use hands under hips for support.

   — Breathe!

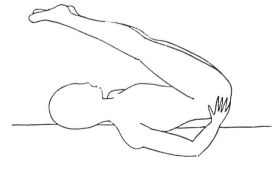

■ SEARCH EXERCISE ANALYSIS TOOL
Hamstring Stretching

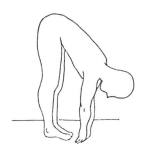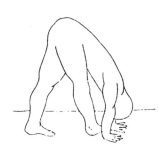

Hamstring Stretching

SEARCH for Exercise Choices Worksheet

DETERMINE IF THE OVERALL PURPOSE OF THE EXERCISE IS TO IMPROVE FLEXIBILITY OR MUSCLE STRENGTH AND ENDURANCE

Complete the section below, checking the appropriate boxes under "Yes," "Maybe," or "No."

FLEXIBILITY

Yes Maybe No

A. Is it important to perform this exercise to counteract the effects of activities of daily life, work, and/or to prepare for recreational pursuits?   ( ) ⊠ ( )

A. While the hamstrings need to be stretched, this position would be discouraged in daily activities such as lifting. This might be a position used in gymnastics and diving.

B. Is the exercise shown and cued in a biomechanically correct way, with possible modifications presented?   ( ) ( ) ⊠

B. Modifications for low back, knees, and blood flow needed.

C. Is there adequate base of support?   ( ) ⊠ ( )

C. The first picture shows a two-point base of support. The second picture shows a four-point base if a person is flexible enough to touch the floor.

D. Does the stretch allow for maximum muscle relaxation and minimization of gravitational pull?   ( ) ( ) ⊠

D. No! The hamstring groups are eccentrically contracting, not stretching, No minimization of gravity is presented.

E. Is this exercise performed using controlled, non-ballistic movements?   ( ) ⊠ ( )

F. Can this exercise be performed *without* compromising other body parts?   ( ) ( ) ⊠

F. The exercises, as shown, would compromise the low back and circulation, especially if performed after aerobic exercise.

Need for Modification - Cuing Tips

1) *Since the exercise is not stretching the hamstring group, the sitting position would minimize gravity and accomplish the goal of stretching the hamstring groups.*

2) *To create a more stable base of support and avoid compromise of low back, go to a sitting position, maintain the low back curve, keep head up, aim chin at feet, use arms for back support.*

3) *The goal is not reaching your toes— the goal is to stretch the hamstring group— this is best accomplished by keeping the knees straight (since this muscle group attaches below the knee).*

4) *Walk hands down to a comfortable stretch and hold. Walk hands up legs to relax.*

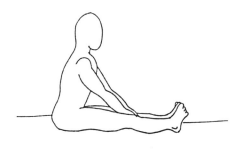

I don't know
what you said,
but I remember
how you said it.
I don't hear a word,
I hear a tone.
I can't recall
if what you said
was important,
but I sure do remember
what you did.

Cindy Herbert
Susan Russell
Every Child's Everyday

Chapter 10

CONCLUSION

■ The majority of us will continue to teach "mixed groups." Our classes will be composed of participants with varying fitness levels, risk factors, attitudes, beliefs, likes, dislikes, and personal needs. We will still be required to lead a group on a fixed schedule and must continue to promote total fitness. We know that our abilities to individualize and modify exercise are important NOW and need to be enlarged to meet the needs of more people, especially those who do not currently exercise.

We hope that you continue to expand your knowledge base. For example, attend workshops on folk or modern dance, stress management, yoga, communication skills, and read the new research in exercise physiology. Consider teaching your own seminars or inservices because you learn more while teaching. Be adventurous! Try new exercise systems such as yoga, the martial arts and sports. Exchange information, newly developed techniques and share music with other educators. Improve. Do not be afraid of change, questions, or how your growth will affect others. This handbook can be used as:

• a starting point, if you are just beginning to explore and teach exercise

• a refreshing review and inspiration for practiced educators

• an information resource and guide

Our society advances toward ever increasing mechanization, therefore, jobs will become increasingly sedentary. Projections for the year 2000 indicate that most of the jobs will require a higher level of education with a decrease in physical labor. For example, as we have entered into the computer/communications age we see a new spectrum of work-related injuries such as carpal tunnel syndrome, CDT exposure, and back injury, not from lifting, but from static positioning. Our job as exercise educators is clear. We will need to continue to assist people in maintaining physical flexibility, muscular strength and endurance, posture, positioning, correct body mechanics, and cardiorespiratory improvement. Moreover, exercise programs will be used increasingly as an adjunct to medical care in the management of stress, pain, addictions, weight control, injury rehabilitation, and cardiopulmonary diseases. We need to continue promoting prevention, active lifestyles, independence and personal self-responsibility.

As an integrated and important part of health maintenance, we will continue to be utilized as a resource on a variety of subjects. The information that we impart will still need to be documented by scientific study rather than by opinion, tradition, hearsay, myth and the "quick fixes" so temptingly offered by advertising. We will continue to confront peoples' value conflicts and together with other health professionals, help resolve them.

Ultimately, however, the value of exercise is not the potential physiological change or increased physical capacity, either of which may be lost to inactivity, disease, or injury. The real enduring value of exercise is personal empowerment, self-image enhancement, social interaction and sharing aspects of our world with others. As exercise educators, we must facilitate this process of growth and nurturing. By example we must promote the concept of lifetime fitness both in and out of our classes. What we do and say in our classes must be consistent. We must treasure and protect these opportunities for our participants and for ourselves. As knowledgeable exercise educators we can make an impact and we do make a difference.

SUGGESTED READING

Aerobics and Fitness Association of America. 1985. *Aerobics Theory and Practice*. Sherman Oaks, California.

Alter, Judith. 1983. *Surviving Exercise*. Boston: Houghton-Mifflin Company.

Alter, Judith. 1986. *Stretch and Strengthen*. Boston: Houghton-Mifflin Company.

Anderson, Bob. 1980. *Stretching*. Bolinas, CA: Shelter Publishers.

Bailey, C. 1989. *The Fit or Fat Woman*. Boston: Houghton-Mifflin Company.

Bouchard, C.; Shephard, R.; Stephens, T.; Sutton, J.; and McPherson, B. 1990. *Exercise, Fitness and Health*. Champaign, IL: Human Kinetics.

Francis, P.; and Francis, L. 1988. *If it Hurts, Don't Do it*. Rocklin, CA: Prima Publishing and Communications.

Golding, L.; Myers, C.; and Sinning, W. 1989. *Y's Way to Physical Fitness*. Champaign, IL: Human Kinetics.

Guyton, A. 1986. *A Textbook of Medical Physiology*. Philadelphia:W.B. Saunders.

Hole, John W. 1981. *Human Anatomy and Physiology*. Dubuque, IA: W.C. Brown Company.

Howley, E.; and Franks, D. *Health/Fitness Instructor's Handbook*. Champaign, IL: Human Kinetics.

IDEA Foundation. 1987. *Aerobic Dance Exercise Instructor Manual*. San Diego, CA.

Kan, Esther. 1987. *Keep It Moving, It's Aerobic Dance*. Mayfield Company.

Kapit, W.; and Elson, L. 1977. *Anatomy Coloring Book*. New York: Harper and Row.

Katch, F.; and McArdle, W. 1988. *Nutrition and Weight Control*. Philadelphia: Lea and Febiger.

Kravitz, Len. 1986. *Anybody's Guide to Total Fitness*. Dubuque, IA: Kendall/Hunt.

Kusinitz, Ivan. 1987. *Your Guide to Getting Fit*. Mayfield Company.

McArdle, W.; Katch, F.; and Katch, V. 1986. *Exercise Physiology, Energy, Nutrition, and Human Performance*. Philadelphia: Lea and Febiger.

McGlynn, G. 1990. *Dynamics of Fitness*. Brown Publishers.

Sharkey, B. 1991. *New Dimensions in Aerobic Fitness*. Champaign, IL: Human Kinetics Publishers.

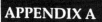

LONG HEALTH HISTORY FORM

Name:_____ Street Address:_____

City, State:_____ Zip Code:_____

Phone Number: Home (_____)_____ Work (_____)_____

Date of Birth:____/____/____ Age:_____ Physician(s):_____

Date of last.....Physical:____/____/____ Surgery:____/____/____ EKG:____/____/____

What, if anything, is your major health problem?_____
_____

Please list any drugs, medication or dietary supplements, PRESCRIBED by a physician, that you are taking now:

Drug:_____ for:_____
Dosage:_____ Reactions:_____

Drug:_____ for:_____
Dosage:_____ Reactions:_____

Please list non-prescription, SELF-PRESCRIBED, medications or supplements that you are taking now:

Drug:_____ for:_____
Dosage:_____ Reactions:_____

Drug:_____ for:_____
Dosage:_____ Reactions:_____

IF NECESSARY, PLEASE LIST OTHER MEDICATIONS ON THE BACK OF THIS PAGE.

PLEASE INDICATE A "YES" RESPONSE TO THE QUESTIONS BELOW BY PLACING A CHECK (✓) IN THE SPACE PROVIDED:

Have you ever been told by a doctor that you have or have had.....

[ ] Rheumatic Fever	[ ] High Blood Cholesterol	[ ] Neck Problems
[ ] Heart Murmur	[ ] High Blood Triglycerides	[ ] Mid-Back Problems
[ ] Heart or Vascular Problems	[ ] Blood Clots/Thrombophlebitis	[ ] Low Back Problems
[ ] High Blood Pressure	[ ] Arthritis	[ ] Varicose Veins
[ ] Heart Attack	[ ] Osteoporosis	[ ] Epilepsy/Seizures
[ ] Heart Failure	[ ] Cancer	[ ] Thyroid Disorders
[ ] Abnormal Electrocardiogram	[ ] Gout or Hyperuricemia	[ ] Diabetes
[ ] Stroke	[ ] Lung or Pulmonary Conditions	[ ] Allergies

Has anyone in your immediate family (grandparents, parents, brothers/sisters) had any of the following?

[ ] Heart Attack or Stroke under age 55	[ ] High Blood Pressure	[ ] Diabetes
[ ] Heart Surgery	[ ] High Blood Cholesterol	[ ] High Blood Triglycerides

Do you smoke?   [ ] NO   [ ] YES.....If yes, how much? [ ] 1/2 pk./day [ ] 1 pk./day [ ] 2 or more pks./day
                                     For how long? [ ] 5 yrs. [ ] 10 yrs. [ ] 15+ yrs.

What type of exercise do you do regularly?

[ ] NONE	[ ] Calisthenics/Floor Exercises	[ ] Outdoor Cycling
[ ] Walking	[ ] Stationary Bicycling	[ ] Weightlifting
[ ] Jogging	[ ] Rebound Trampoline	[ ] Dancing
[ ] Running	[ ] Competitive Sports	[ ] Swimming/Aquatic Exercise
[ ] Other:_____		

How many times per week do you participate in the activities listed above?

(Please circle)   1   2   3   4   5   6   7

How much time do you spend at each session?   [ ] less than 15 minutes;

[ ] 15-20 min.   [ ] 20-30 min.   [ ] 30-45 min.   [ ] 45-60 min.   [ ] 60 min.+

What word best describes how hard your average workout is?

[ ] Very Light   [ ] Light   [ ] Moderate   [ ] Hard   [ ] Very Hard   [ ] Extremely Hard

While exercising, with exertion, or after exercise – do you experience.....

[ ] Shortness of breath or wheezing	[ ] Nausea	[ ] Overall/1-sided weakness	[ ] Fainting
[ ] Side aches or side stitches	[ ] Dizziness	[ ] Mental confusion	[ ] Vomiting
[ ] Extremely high heart rate	[ ] Back pain	[ ] Sharp chest pain	[ ] Heat intolerance
[ ] Irregular pulse or palpitations	[ ] Muscle cramping	[ ] Dull, aching chest pain	[ ] Arm or neck pain
[ ] Swelling of ankles or hands	[ ] Shin splints	[ ] Ankle or foot pain	[ ] Knee or hip pain
[ ] Extreme lasting pain or fatigue	[ ] Calf pain	[ ] Lack of coordination	[ ] Shoulder pain

What would you like to accomplish through exercise?_____

I acknowledge that my answers to the questions are true and complete. I will immediately inform the exercise instructor of any changes in my health.

Signature:_____ Date:_____

SHORT HEALTH HISTORY AND CONSENT FORM

Name:_____ Date:_____

The following information will be kept strictly confidential and will only be utilized to make the exercise portions of this workshop or class safe. Please check any conditions that may apply to you.

Have you ever been told by a physician that you have or have had:

[ ] Heart attack   [ ] High cholesterol levels (>200)   [ ] Cancer   [ ] Arthritis
[ ] Seizures   [ ] High Blood Pressure   [ ] Diabetes   [ ] Osteoporosis
[ ] Stroke   [ ] Abnormal EKG   [ ] Lung problems   [ ] Gout

If you are currently taking any PRESCRIPTION OR OVER-THE-COUNTER medications, please list:

_____

_____

Do you smoke?   [ ] YES   [ ] NO   Can you swim?   [ ] YES   [ ] NO (for an aquatics class only)

Do you exercise, aerobically, at least 3-4 times/week?   [ ] YES   [ ] NO

Do you have any past injuries to, or current problems with, any of the areas listed:

[ ] Irregular heart beat   [ ] Dizziness   [ ] Neck   [ ] Low back   [ ] Feet
[ ] Chest pain   [ ] Fainting   [ ] Hands   [ ] Mid-back   [ ] Ankles
[ ] Loss of coordination   [ ] Cramping   [ ] Hips   [ ] Shoulders   [ ] Knees
[ ] Heat intolerance   [ ] Shin splints   [ ] Calves

I realize that there are risks to ALL exercise, including injury and possible death. While every effort will be made to decrease any risk of injury, I take full responsibility for my participation in this class. Knowing that I may participate at my own pace, and that I am free to discontinue participation at any time, I will inform the instructor/workshop leader of any problems – immediately.

Signature:_____ Date:_____

SHORT HEALTH HISTORY AND CONSENT FORM

Name:_____ Date:_____

The following information will be kept strictly confidential and will only be utilized to make the exercise portions of this workshop or class safe. Please check any conditions that may apply to you.

Have you ever been told by a physician that you have or have had:

[ ] Heart attack   [ ] High cholesterol levels (>200)   [ ] Cancer   [ ] Arthritis
[ ] Seizures   [ ] High Blood Pressure   [ ] Diabetes   [ ] Osteoporosis
[ ] Stroke   [ ] Abnormal EKG   [ ] Lung problems   [ ] Gout

If you are currently taking any PRESCRIPTION OR OVER-THE-COUNTER medications, please list:

_____

_____

Do you smoke?   [ ] YES   [ ] NO   Can you swim?   [ ] YES   [ ] NO (for an aquatics class only)

Do you exercise, aerobically, at least 3-4 times/week?   [ ] YES   [ ] NO

Do you have any past injuries to, or current problems with, any of the areas listed:

[ ] Irregular heart beat   [ ] Dizziness   [ ] Neck   [ ] Low back   [ ] Feet
[ ] Chest pain   [ ] Fainting   [ ] Hands   [ ] Mid-back   [ ] Ankles
[ ] Loss of coordination   [ ] Cramping   [ ] Hips   [ ] Shoulders   [ ] Knees
[ ] Heat intolerance   [ ] Shin splints   [ ] Calves

I realize that there are risks to ALL exercise, including injury and possible death. While every effort will be made to decrease any risk of injury, I take full responsibility for my participation in this class. Knowing that I may participate at my own pace, and that I am free to discontinue participation at any time, I will inform the instructor/workshop leader of any problems – immediately.

Signature:_____ Date:_____

INFORMED CONSENT FORM – EXERCISE PARTICIPATION

I desire to engage <u>voluntarily</u> in _____ in order to improve my physical fitness.   (name of program, club, or agency)

I know that I am required to fill out a health and lifestyle questionnaire <u>before</u> I begin to exercise. The information obtained from the questionnaire will be utilized to:

1)   Indicate any <u>cardiac risk</u> or <u>other reason why I should not exercise</u>.
2)   Determine the need for a physician's <u>evaluation and/or written approval</u> before entering the exercise program.
3)   Recommend the <u>types of exercise</u> I should concentrate on to reach my fitness goals and types of exercises I should avoid.

I understand that my participation in the program may <u>NOT</u> benefit me directly in any way. I realize that the program <u>may help me evaluate my lifestyle, those activities I may safely carry out, and may increase the quality of my present lifestyle</u>.

I also understand that the reaction of the body to activity cannot always be predicted with complete accuracy. The changes that may occur and are associated with physical activity include, but are not limited to these signs and symptoms: <u>ABNORMAL BLOOD PRESSURE OR HEART RATE RESPONSES, BREATHLESSNESS, CHEST DISCOMFORT, MUSCULAR OR SKELETAL INJURY AND, IN VERY RARE INSTANCES, HEART ATTACK AND DEATH</u>. I realize <u>my</u> responsibility in recognizing these potential hazards, monitoring myself before, during and after exercise and seeking help in the event of injury, if possible. I will attend the orientation session and talk to my personal trainer or exercise instructor, to learn how to minimize these potential hazards and what I should do in an emergency. I understand that <u>I can take steps to minimize my risk</u> during exercise by following the steps noted below:

1)   I will give priority to <u>regular attendance</u>.
2)   I will <u>not withhold any information</u> pertinent to my health or condition to the instructor/supervisor in charge of the program, and will <u>immediately update</u> my health and lifestyle questionnaire if changes in medication or status should occur.
3)   I will <u>report any unusual symptom or problem</u> that I experience before, during, or after exercise.
4)   I will <u>follow the amounts and types</u> of activities recommended during the orientation session.
5)   I will <u>not exceed</u> my target heart rate.
6)   I will <u>not exercise</u> when <u>not feeling well</u> or for <u>2 hours after eating</u>, after <u>smoking</u> a cigarette, after <u>drinking alcohol</u>, or <u>taking over-the-counter medications or "street" drugs</u>.
7)   I will <u>cool down</u> slowly after exercise, and will <u>not take</u> an <u>extremely hot</u> shower after exercise.
8)   I will <u>not</u> undertake <u>isometric, straining</u>, or any other exercise I know by experience or my physician's or therapist's recommendation, to be <u>painful or detrimental</u> to me.
9)   I realize that <u>unsupervised exercise</u> done on my own is <u>performed at my own risk</u>, even though I may be following guidelines or recommendations established during this program.

The information obtained from this exercise program will be treated as <u>privileged and confidential</u>, and will not be released to any person without my written consent. Information regarding my health and program may be shared with instructors involved in my instruction or physical training. The information obtained may also be used for statistical or scientific purposes, with my right to privacy retained.

I, the undersigned, waive and release _____, its employees,   (name of program, club, or agency)
officers or directors, against any and all claims in any way connected with my participation in this program. This agreement is binding on my heirs and executors.

I acknowledge that I have <u>read or heard</u> this document in its entirety and that I fully understand it. Any questions which may have occurred to me have been <u>asked</u> by me and have been <u>answered</u> to my satisfaction.

_____   _____   _____   _____
Signature   Date   Witness   Date